Jessica Maguire has a Bachelor of Health Science and a Master of Physiotherapy. Her post-graduate study has included work in neuroscience, neuroplasticity, neurology, brain–heart biofeedback, modern pain science, and transcutaneous vagus nerve stimulation.

A TEDx speaker and lecturer, she believes that knowledge is power. Jessica has taught thousands of students from all over the world to transform their nervous system, empowering them to step into the driver's seat of their own health and wellbeing.

Her mission is to widen the world's collective window of tolerance, and to create true freedom from nervous system dysregulation and all its painful side effects.

The NERVOUS SYSTEM RESET

Heal Trauma, Resolve Chronic Stress and Pain, and Regulate Your Emotions with the Power of the Vagus Nerve

JESSICA MAGUIRE

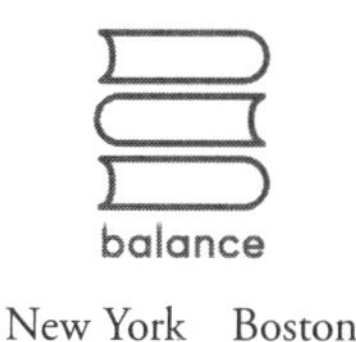

New York Boston

Balance
Hachette Book Group
1290 Avenue of the Americas
New York, NY 10104
GCP-Balance.com
@GCPBalance

Originally published in 2024 in Australia by Pan Macmillan Australia Pty Ltd
First US edition: August 2024

Balance is an imprint of Grand Central Publishing. The Balance name and logo are registered trademarks of Hachette Book Group, Inc.

Illustrations on pages 22, 73, 75, 84, 86, 96, 101, 144, 146, 149, 150, and 294 by Jake Milton
Image on page 72 by Schappelle, CC BY-SA 4.0
Images on pages 107, 113, 114, 125, and 228 from Shutterstock

Library of Congress Cataloging-in-Publication Data has been applied for.

ISBNs: 9781538757123 (hardcover), 9781538757147 (ebook)

Printed in Canada

MRQ-T

Printing 1, 2024

For Ivy and Sam

Contents

INTRODUCTION
I think I know why you're here

Something feels 'off' in your body, heart and mind, and you're searching for information to ease your physical or emotional distress. You may have spent a year or more cycling through appointments with various healthcare professionals to address these issues, and even had bloodwork or other lab tests done in an effort to get to the bottom of whatever's going on. You've probably trialled one or more medications and/or supplement regimes, and I bet you've exhausted Google looking for answers.

Am I on the right track? If I am, it's because I've seen these scenarios play out hundreds of times over the many years I've been guiding people through their healing journey – first as a physiotherapist, and now as a leading global educator on the nervous system. I understand how hard it is to stay positive and afloat in this sea of uncertainty, and I've seen how living with chronic health problems without an obvious cause or solution can bring people to the brink of despair and even make them wonder if the problem is all in their head.

Does this sound like you?

By the time people come to me for help, they're usually tired, in pain and emotionally drained from months, years or even decades of an uphill health battle. Alex was one of these patients.

Alex's story: Restoring balance

My first impression of Alex was that she was full of life and a perfectly healthy 31-year-old, but a few minutes of conversation changed my mind. Alex had lived with ongoing health issues since the age of 25. Initially, she suffered with severe skin irritation in her twenties, but before long she was also dealing with pain in her stomach, along with anxiety and a cluster of other conditions, each requiring different treatments. Over the years, Alex had seen dozens of doctors and been prescribed a litany of medications – so many she could hardly remember them all.

Some of Alex's doctors had hypothesised that her skin condition was a result of irritation from cosmetics and other products, so she dutifully switched to the creams they prescribed and changed every product she used, from her soap to her laundry detergent. When that didn't help, other doctors wondered if she was causing ongoing irritation by scratching her arms without realising it – perhaps in her sleep or while worrying about something. Though Alex was adamant she hadn't been doing this, their best advice was for her to make an effort not to touch the affected areas at all, and then see if anything changed. It didn't.

All of this was very frustrating, and didn't help soothe the itchiness, pain or appearance of the red blotches that covered her arms. She grew increasingly self-conscious about her skin and started dreading going to work. If a colleague or friend happened to mention her skin in any way, she became angry and defensive.

When her body aches, stomach pain and digestive issues cropped up, Alex was diagnosed with irritable bowel syndrome (IBS) and prescribed a strict diet. Despite following that diet to the letter, her symptoms continued unchecked. With no relief, she resorted to reorganising her life around her stomach pain – avoiding social occasions and dinners with friends in case a rogue ingredient caused a flare-up.

While dealing with these health challenges, Alex developed anxiety, which worsened despite visits to specialists and various prescriptions. As I took her history, I noticed that she described herself as 'a worry wart' and 'an anxious person'. This was an important detail, because it gave me a lot of insight into the stories Alex was telling about herself. She obviously believed that these descriptions of herself were accurate, because she stated them as factually as she'd reported her experience of physical pain.

Alex characterising herself in this way – as a 'worrier' – was contributing to a lack of trust in herself. Despite all she'd been through, I was starting to wonder if her anxious nature was leading her brain to sound alarms that amplified her pain.

What *was* clear to me, though, was that Alex's conditions were not only very real, but had also gone unvalidated and unseen for years. That lack of support and validation had, in turn, created the perfect environment for other issues to arise. I've listened to many patients and students describe mental and physical pain, and express disillusionment with medical approaches and various mindset practices they've been advised to try. Many have been told that their symptoms are either psychosomatic or 'not that bad'.

Others have been assured that talking about their suffering and mindfulness will cure them, and then been frustrated when they've pursued those strategies without any improvement. While these are both good interventions in certain situations, in Alex's case they were only treating the visible *symptoms* rather than the root of her pain.

After I'd taken a thorough case history from Alex, she confided that it hadn't just been her skin condition that had first led to her anxiety developing. Around the same time she sought treatment for her skin, she'd also had a major blow-up with her housemate. For months, Alex had been coming home from work to find piles of her housemate's dishes in the sink and clutter in the living room. Initially, she'd tried ignoring the mess, hoping her housemate would take the hint, but when they didn't, she started cleaning up after them – though doing so made her furious. After months of doing this without so much as a thank you, Alex sat her housemate down and told them things had to change – but they didn't seem very interested in changing.

This situation went on for well over a year, but when Alex had to cover her housemate's late rent payment for the second time, she'd finally had enough and confronted her housemate. They'd argued, but the housemate had eventually apologised and promised to do better. When Alex got home from work the next day, however, her housemate was gone and so was all of their stuff. Though Alex was relieved not to be living with them any more, it put her in a tough spot financially. She maxed out her credit card covering the extra rent and bills while she scrambled to find a new housemate. She felt helpless about her financial situation and at times she'd felt a sense of panic, knowing that she simply couldn't cover the cost and there was a current rental shortage in her area.

This information was the missing piece of the puzzle for me, and I felt confident that nervous system dysregulation had not only triggered the inflammatory response that had caused Alex's skin condition, but was also behind many of the health problems she was currently experiencing.

Our internal thermostat and set point

Every one of us has an internal set point at which we feel and function our best. Like a thermostat in a house, our brain and body work together via our nervous system to bring us back to our set point and maintain this beautiful equilibrium – or what scientists call homeostasis.

Ideally, we'd spend the majority of our lives thriving at this comfortable set point, but it's not the only setting on our internal thermostat. There are two others – hot and cold – and both are necessary – even life-saving in certain circumstances. We're wired to slip in and out of these two quickly as life demands. If we're under attack, for example, switching to a hotter state allows us to react quickly and with aggression to defend ourselves or to run away. This is colloquially known as fight or flight. In a well-regulated system, once the threat has passed we come back to our set point and return to our lives.

The remarkable thing about this set point is that it's calibrated to meet our *true* needs (i.e. the needs of our lived reality). Unfortunately, factors such as illness, trauma and chronic stress can swing us away from this set point, and even change it entirely.

If we exist in a hot or cold state for long enough for our brain to perceive it as our new reality, our set point will recalibrate to meet what it *believes* to be our true needs. Our brain is a 'prediction machine' and if we've experienced traumatic stress and become hypervigilant to threat, our set point may shift so that it's calibrated to our *predicted* needs (how we perceive our reality).

In Alex's case, the stress of living with an inconsiderate housemate had dialled her thermostat up to a hotter temperature. And after months of her swallowing her irritation, anger and stress, Alex's thermostat had decided that this hotter temperature was her new normal, and had adjusted her set point accordingly. The final straw was the helplessness she felt of not being able to find a housemate and being left with the responsibility of paying rent that was more than she could afford.

If we want to feel good and perform at our best, the most powerful thing we can do is recalibrate what's going on inside our body and brain, to match the real demands of our environment.

Just imagine how uncomfortable it would be to live in a house where the thermostat was stuck on an extreme temperature. Your mood, not to mention your capacity to deal with stress would be radically altered. Every task would require more effort and energy – you'd either have to keep a fire burning constantly and wear extra clothing to stay warm, or find ways to stay cool in the stifling heat.

Left unchecked, those extreme temperatures start to cause short-term emergencies. Hardwood floors start to buckle or crack in the heat. Pipes freeze and burst in the cold and, just like that, the ongoing temperature problem becomes an all-out emergency – draining precious resources and distracting you from the routine maintenance projects that keep your house running smoothly.

A similar type of wear and tear goes on inside us. Yes, we can handle certain situations and environments in the short term, such as staying up all night to meet a work deadline, or being a 24-hour caregiver for an ill family member over a couple of weeks. But when we push past our natural limits to meet expectations or please others, our body sends us warning signs to let us know we're shifting away from our set-point. The longer we stay in those situations and the more we yield to the pervasive cultural pressure to be busy, work hard and achieve more, the more we overstep our natural limits, the further we get from that healthy, regulated set point, and the worse we feel. Regulation turns into dysregulation and, over time, this manifests as mental and/or physical conditions we can no longer ignore.

Stress, trauma and our shifting baseline

Like so many of our feelings, emotions and experiences, stress and trauma exist on a spectrum, and while all trauma is stressful, not all stress is traumatic. Stress refers to the way our brain and body respond to an event or situation we perceive as threatening or challenging. As we all know, stress can be mild or major. Everyday stressors are rarely threats to our survival, but our brain doesn't usually realise that. In the face of stress, we're hardwired to mobilise energy and trigger stress-arousal responses.

These hardwired fight-or-flight responses prepare us for danger by turning up the temperature on our set point, but if the stress is only mild, it sharpens our focus and mobilises our energy so we're ready for action. And just as we're designed to cope with stressful moments, a process known as ***allostasis*** **gives us the capacity to return to our baseline once that threat has passed.** It's a process of mobilising energy to meet demands and then completing that stress activation cycle. With a healthy, functioning nervous system, we can return to a calm state where we feel social and at ease fairly quickly. Provided we get to recover fully from stress, it's not bad for us. In fact, in most cases it makes us more resilient.

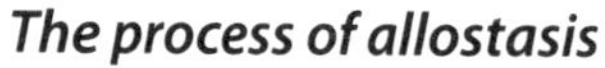

The process of allostasis

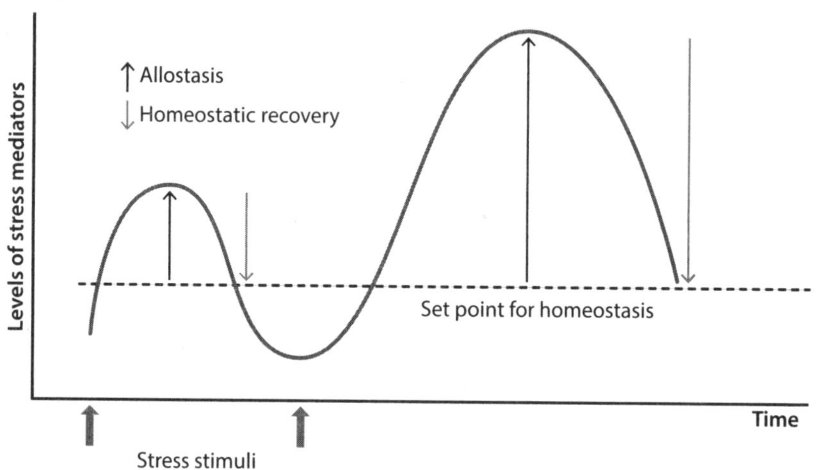

But when stress is chronic and we experience panic or anxiety on an ongoing basis, it depletes our resources and energy and takes a toll on our body. The wear and tear caused by this cumulative stress is known as *allostatic load*, and it can contribute to physical ailments such as digestive disorders and hypertension, as well as mental health issues such as depression. The important consequence of allostatic load is that it can prevent us from returning to our original set point. The same is true of traumatic stress, which occurs when we experience too much stress, too quickly.

The effect of allostatic load

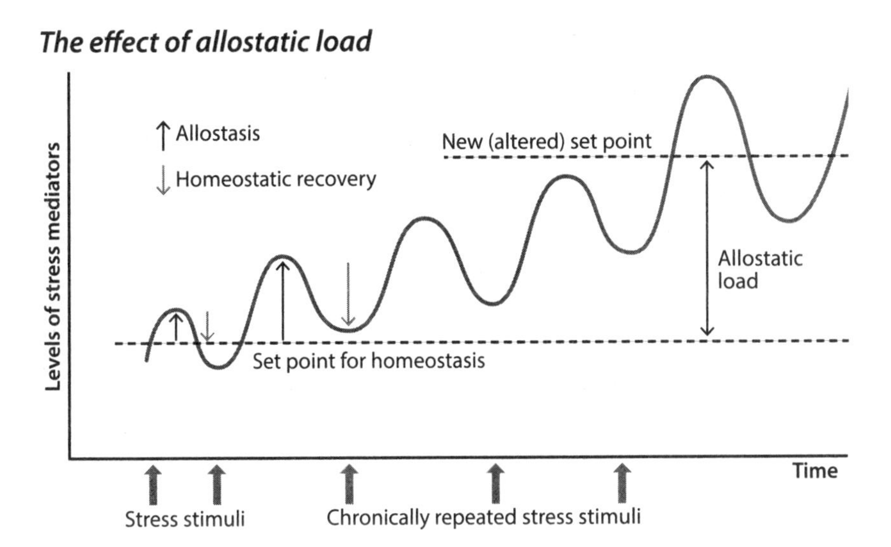

Cortisol gets a bad rap for being the 'stress hormone', but it performs the vital job of mobilising glucose so we have the energy we need to meet challenges. Prolonged periods of stress can cause fluctuations in our cortisol levels, and this can lead to burnout, an increasingly common condition, as too little cortisol leaves us feeling flat, unmotivated and fatigued. When we spend a long time feeling depleted like this, our nervous system can shift even further into that 'too cold' state, and this can lead to feeling flat, numb and depressed. Crucially, this can also change our inner thermostat and recalibrate our set point to a lower temperature.

At the other end of the spectrum is *trauma*, which ranges from extreme ongoing stress to highly distressing events. Like stress, trauma can recalibrate our set point. It's important to note that there's no one point on this continuum where stress crosses the line into trauma. This is because trauma is subjective and context matters. Our individual history (especially events that are similar), personality, beliefs, values and genetics inform what our idea of trauma is and how we experience it. What's traumatic for one person may be only annoying to another.

We can also understand trauma as an experience (or several experiences) that overwhelms our capacity to regulate our emotions and bodily sensations, and make sense of the world and our own experience. It leads to a fragmentation, a *dissociation* that can cause us to feel disconnected from our body, and lead to a dysregulation of our nervous system and our emotions, making it hard for our body to control or regulate our mood and emotional responses.

Trauma is not about a past event, but about our present experience and the reaction we're still having in our brain and our body today.

Stress and trauma scale

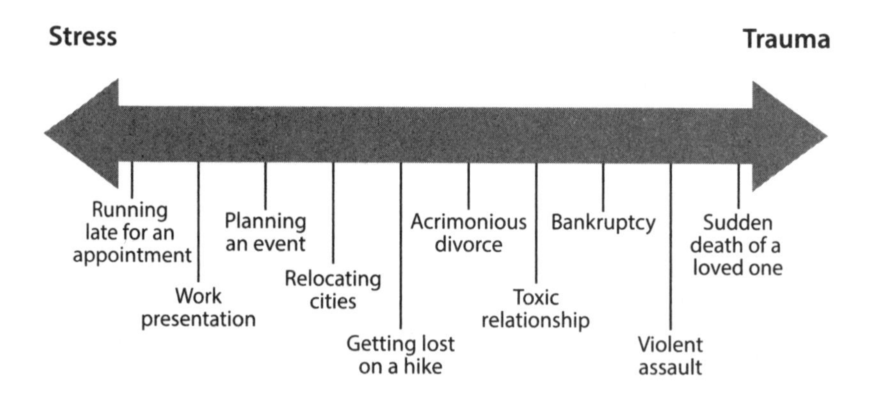

The exact point at which we label or judge our stress, or an experience, as traumatic is less important than recognising and healing the dysregulation that lives on in our brain and body. Dysregulation can spread beyond our nervous system to the many systems it communicates closely with, including our immune, endocrine, cardiovascular, musculoskeletal and digestive systems.

Alex's story: Stuck in the hot state

In Alex's case, the stress she was experiencing at home was causing her to spend too much time in her hotter, more activated state. This impacted her immune system, which caused the inflammatory response in her skin. Worries about what was causing her skin condition resulted in Alex's racing thoughts, which led her to become anxious and, eventually, irritable.

With no relief from the source of stress at home, these ongoing stress responses triggered changes in Alex's sensitive digestive system. The IBS symptoms Alex began to experience, coupled with a lack of effective support from the health practitioners she was paying to see, only compounded her dysregulation. Nervous system dysregulation is a lot like the iceberg illustrated overleaf. The unpleasant behaviour, actions and responses we see in ourselves and others are visible on the surface. These side effects on the surface might also manifest as seemingly isolated conditions with no clear root cause. For many, these conditions persist for years, creating knock-on effects in their health and life that lead to *more* discomfort and unhappiness, further decreasing their quality of life. Below the surface, however, there's a lot more going on, and if we don't dive under the water to tackle those root causes of our physical, emotional or mental distress, we're destined to keep putting band-aids over bullet holes.

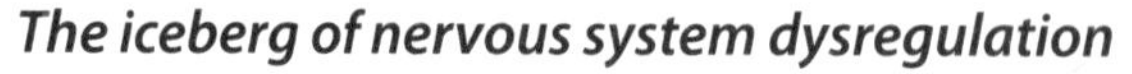

The iceberg of nervous system dysregulation

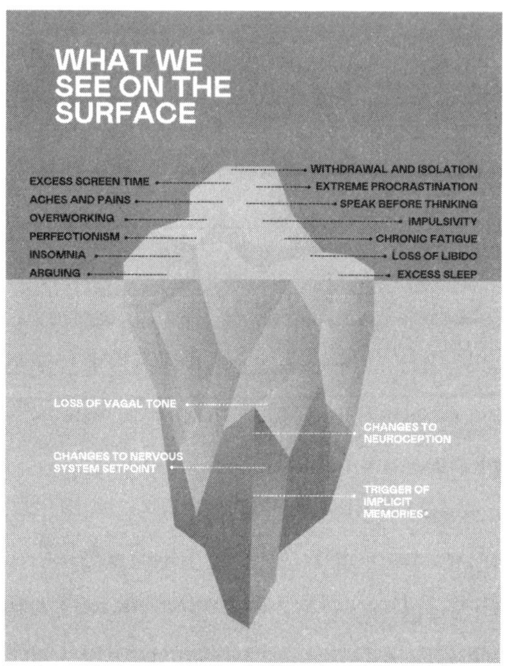

Typically, those band-aids take the form of 'artificial regulators', such as alcohol, comfort food, sugar, caffeine, excessive social media use or online gaming, TV, stimulants or pharmaceutical medication. We know that we don't like how we feel, so we reach for something to make us feel 'better', but relief and regulation are only short term because they don't address the true root cause, which is a dysregulated nervous system.

To start with, I asked Alex to pay attention to both her emotions and her bodily signals, such as changes in her posture, when she found herself worrying about her health or her finances. When I speak about posture here it's not the 'stand up straight' kind of posture. This is the habitual ways the body braces, collapses or freezes when we feel threatened. I wanted her to experience that there's no real separation between our brain and our body. It's why 'brain–body connection' (or the 'brain–body system', as I like to call it) is such an important part of understanding how trauma can lead to things like gut disorders and persistent pain.

The standard biomedical model

Despite the widely accepted connection between the brain and the body – for example, psychosomatic illnesses have been recognised for centuries – since the twentieth century the *biomedical model* has become the dominant approach to treating physical pain and distress. This focuses on biological processes and physiology, and in many cases it works well. After all, in the right circumstances, many diseases, infections and ailments *can* be treated in isolation and cured or alleviated by medications or surgical interventions.

But since the biomedical approach centres predominantly on the patient's biology at the moment of examination rather than the factors that played into causing the ailment in the first place, this model can't reliably make sense of (or therefore resolve) some chronic conditions that can arise from nervous system dysregulation – a change in our set point – such as gut issues, inflammatory conditions, skin irritation, hypertension and persistent pain.

Similarly, when we experience *emotional* suffering or our behaviour changes, we might turn to Google for more information, think through how we'll handle a situation we're anxious about – to the point of it keeping us awake at night – or lean on mindset resources to bring us back into balance. These strategies will most likely be 'head-based' approaches geared to helping us *think* our way to wellness. But when we're overwhelmed or facing a crisis, simply reframing what's happening, challenging our mindset or thinking positively is very unlikely to pull us out of that state, because there's so much more going on behind the scenes than we realise.

Our bodies simply can't be talked out of feeling danger. Positive talk may get us some of the way there, but without understanding our neurobiology and tackling the reasons we're experiencing those overwhelming sensations in the first place, our bodies stay stuck in danger mode. Though some head-based approaches do touch on the importance of the brain–body connection, most fail to harness the power of the mind to change overwhelming bodily sensations. Because of that, few of us walk away with any real understanding of what this connection feels like, how it works or how drastically it can impact every aspect of our lives. It's time for us to change this.

The biopsychosocial model: A holistic approach

If you're just beginning to learn about the nervous system, it might come as a shock to find out how much our bodily signals and internal organs impact how we *feel* and how we *think*, but they do. As Alex discovered through our work together, our thoughts, beliefs, emotions and expectations have the power to positively or negatively impact our biological functioning and even how we hold our body. Those same thoughts, beliefs and emotions are even powerful enough to trigger and maintain physical pain.

In this book, we'll be taking a more 'whole person' approach to regulation, known as the *biopsychosocial model*. Unlike the biomedical model, this approach not only fully embraces the two-way relationship between the brain and body, but also takes into account the many ways that our environment, experiences and relationships affect this system. It's premised on the idea that in order to understand our health, we must look at more than just our biology. We must also consider how we're doing mentally and emotionally, and what our social environment looks like, because all three factors are always in play and cannot be separated.

The path to regulation isn't body *or* brain, it's body *and* brain.

The biopsychosocial model

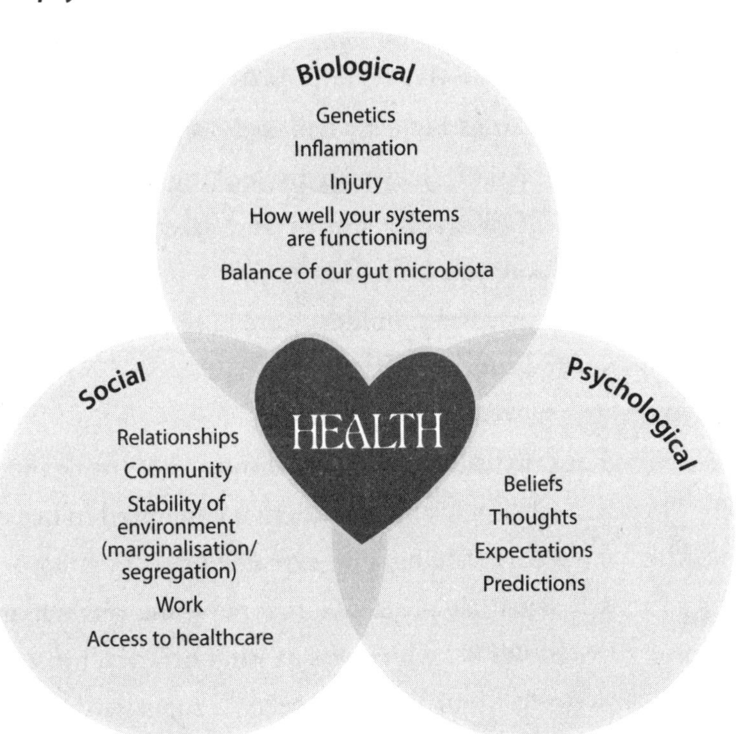

Lisa's story: The biopsychosocial model in action

To better understand how powerful this approach can be, let's look at another one of my patients, Lisa, through this lens. Lisa came to me for treatment of lower back pain and anxiety. Right away, I noticed that the range of movement in her spine was very limited. She braced herself in anticipation of pain when sitting down, and when speaking she spoke quickly and took shallow breaths. When I asked Lisa if I could assess her spine by having her bend over a little, she was resistant. 'What do you think will happen if you bend forwards?' I asked.

'Mum had a herniated disc, too, and her doctor said that bending forwards might make it slip further.'

'Do you have a herniated disc?' I asked, confused. That diagnosis hadn't been in the files from her doctor.

'Well, nothing showed up on the MRI of my lower back, so I think the problem must be really bad and deep.'

'In that case,' I said, 'let's start by looking at your posture.' I had her stand in front of a mirror and asked, 'What do you notice about the way you hold your body?'

Lisa observed that her shoulders were raised, but she brushed this off immediately, saying that she'd always stood this way. She'd noticed this in photos of her as a child.

I pointed out that she was bracing through her trunk and that there was excess tension in the muscles that connected to her spine even when she wasn't moving, and explained that by holding her body so tensely – in that protective manner – she was making it harder to move her spine, which was causing her even more pain.

'See if you can let your shoulders relax,' I suggested. 'That will help you breathe more fully, because when you breathe from your upper chest rather than from your diaphragm, you can only take shallow breaths, and this breathing pattern can influence your nervous system in negative ways.'

We also discussed one important factor that can affect the development of ongoing pain and disability in people with lower back pain: their beliefs about their pain. I noted that Lisa believed that because her mother had persistent back pain, she was destined to have the same condition.

In subsequent sessions, we worked with her spine on a physical level, but also explored the wider context of her life. Lisa noted that the pain in her lower back had started shortly after her relationship with her partner ended. Around that same time, she also got a new boss she felt uncomfortable around. Something about him rubbed her up the wrong way, and she felt quite reactive even when he asked her harmless questions. Around him, she said she felt like she 'had to get out of the office'.

I taught Lisa a few techniques to help calm her nervous system down, which would help to relax her muscles. With repeated practise, her shoulders dropped, her face softened, and her breath became fuller. With time, she was even able to bend and move her back without experiencing excruciating pain.

Over her next few visits, I explained to Lisa that her pain was very real and it wasn't 'all in her head'. I also explained that pain doesn't always equal tissue damage. Sometimes, pain gets worse when we're anxious because it's our body's way of protecting us. Lisa and I spent time trying to understand why her boss, in particular, made her feel so uneasy. Then she happened to mention that he looked like the man who'd married her mother not long after her father's death. As a child, she'd felt on edge, nervous, and scared around her stepfather. He was intimidating and could be cruel, so she avoided him. The way her body was responding to her new boss in the present day was very similar, because the fear and powerlessness felt familiar.

Intellectually, Lisa knew there was no reason to fear her new boss, but her 'survival brain' – the primitive part of our brain that's focused on keeping us alive and protecting us from danger – believed otherwise, and the bodily responses it was sending were making her anxious. Chronic and traumatic stress not only influence the nervous system but also immune responses, which may amplify pain through a number of brain–body system pathways, such as inflammation.

This was a major breakthrough, and we determined that the real work that needed to be done was not solely physiotherapy or trialling new medications to help ease the pain, it was training her brain and body to come out of survival mode; so that it wasn't being overprotective and she could return to a state of regulation and reduce both her physical and emotional pain. Recent research has confirmed that emotion regulation is a successful intervention in reducing persistent pain.

Lisa's case through a biopsychosocial lens

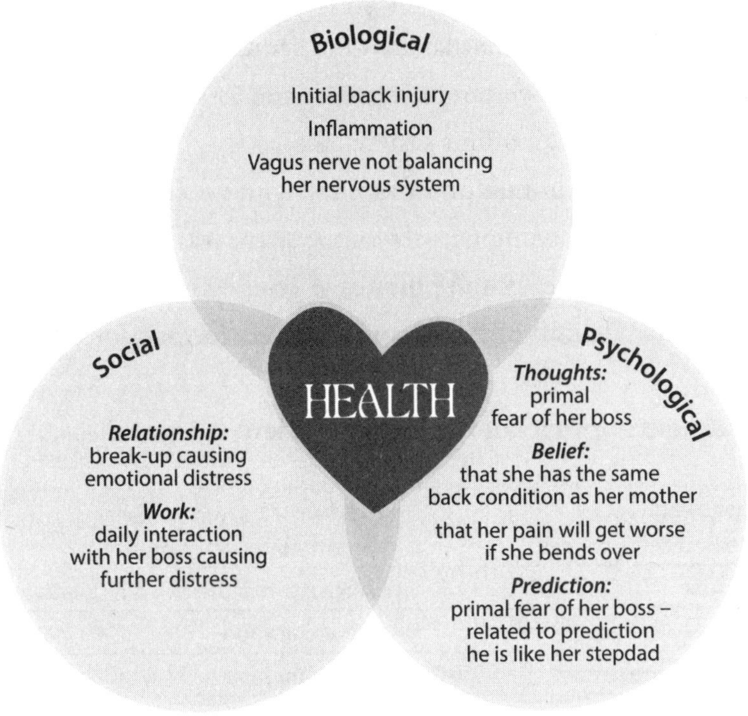

Biological

Initial back injury

Inflammation

Vagus nerve not balancing her nervous system

Social

Relationship: break-up causing emotional distress

Work: daily interaction with her boss causing further distress

HEALTH

Psychological

Thoughts: primal fear of her boss

Belief: that she has the same back condition as her mother

that her pain will get worse if she bends over

Prediction: primal fear of her boss – related to prediction he is like her stepdad

The nervous system dysregulation caused by Lisa's primal fear of her boss not only led to poorly regulated emotional responses, but actually caused inflammation in her body, which then drove more anxiety. This is an example of what can happen when our *neuroimmune system* – i.e. our nervous system *and* our immune system – is disrupted.

Because of the way sciences have been set up to compartmentalise and study each physical system in isolation, the immune system has been seen as a self-regulating entity that works away quietly in the background for our benefit. Immunology has even become a specialised field largely independent of other disciplines.

But immunologists have now realised that our immune system isn't actually self-regulated – it works closely with the nervous system at many different levels. Our neuroimmune system influences how we recover from injuries, and is another example of how intertwined all of our systems are.

For Lisa, inflammation, combined with the fact that her vagus nerve wasn't balancing her nervous system, was driving how bad she felt both mentally and physically. To effectively treat her pain, we had to tackle all of the factors that were feeding into it.

Treatment approaches to Lisa's condition

Past treatments – biomedical approach	What we tried – biopsychological approach
Exercise	Exercise with a friend (co-regulation)
Pain medication	Pain medication
Avoiding movement	Manual therapy
Surgery	Talk therapy
Anti-inflammatories	Pain and nervous system education
Injections	Gentle yoga

It's worth noting that dysregulation is amplified when we feel powerless. This is why autonomy and agency are such powerful antidotes. That all-important sense of autonomy and agency comes from learning to read our internal thermostat settings with greater accuracy, and trusting that we can recognise when our inner environment is changing so we can deploy the appropriate tools to remain in balance. When we feel safe, our body optimises itself for health, growth and restoration. But when we feel unsafe, it triggers defense systems that impair this.

In the end, the thing that made the most difference to Lisa's situation was spending more time in a regulated state. We achieved this through using specific tools for nervous system regulation and her learning to recognise her own nervous system responses. Building this awareness of what was happening in her body and *why* it was happening not only cultivated emotional regulation and reduced Lisa's anxiety, but it also improved her physical health. Her posture improved; her muscular tension diminished, especially in her shoulders and spine; and her mobility increased. By bringing herself back to regulation, Lisa managed to significantly decrease the pain that had been lowering her quality of life for so many years.

The vagus nerve: An introduction

Taking a biopsychosocial approach isn't about 'hacking' or bypassing what's happening in our body, it's about learning to attune ourselves to what's happening in our brain–body system and using this information to shape how we actively take care of our emotional state and our physiology. This could be as simple as noticing the sensations of thirst and having a drink of water, or acknowledging the relentless anxiety we feel about our work and being honest with ourselves that something needs to change. This is how we can achieve true regulation and improve the quality of our life, health, emotional wellbeing and relationships.

The route to engaging and working with all three areas of the biopsychosocial model – our biology, psychology and social interactions – is via an incredible structure called the vagus nerve, a major nerve that connects our brain with our most important systems, via our neck, chest, heart and lungs, to our gut. Once you've read this book, you'll know what the vagus nerve is, how it functions and how to strengthen it. And that will allow you to address so many problems at their source. This is because a dysregulated nervous system can be responsible for a host of chronic health issues, from anxiety, depression and burnout to IBS, some autoimmune disorders and persistent pain.

Image of vagus nerve in body

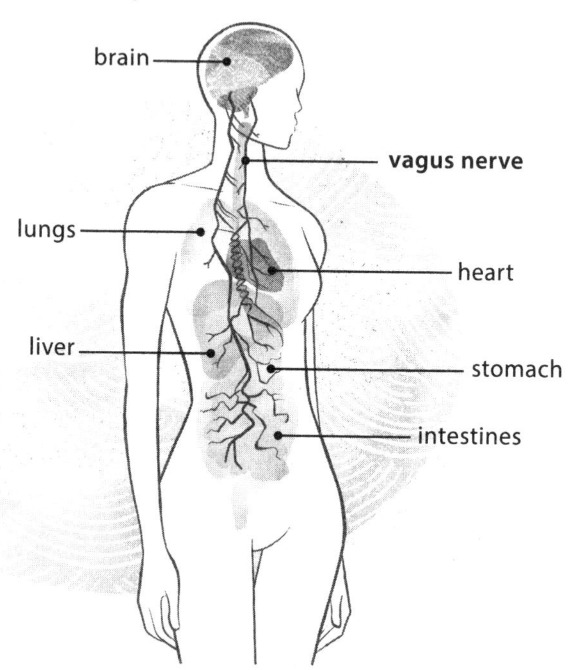

Engaging the vagus nerve is a skill that can be taught, and though we're dealing with training a nerve rather than a muscle, this process is called increasing *vagal tone*. In the same way we can tone muscle through training and exercise, we can improve the function of our vagus nerve by building vagal tone. Resetting your nervous system is going to depend on this, because it's your vagus nerve that brings you to regulation. It's the major part of the nervous system that speeds us up or slows us back down. This in turn leads to better health and a calmer, more balanced state of being. To say the vagus nerve is hugely important is an understatement, and that's why we'll explore its many functions in greater depth in Part One. For now, just know that it's a doorway to emotional, mental and physical wellbeing

I'm not advocating that we throw out the biomedical model – far from it. I still believe that it's essential for medical professionals to rule out organic issues before putting it down to nervous system imbalances, but it's equally important to recognise that many 'medically unexplained symptoms' may well be rooted in a stress-related disorder. For too long, the bodily manifestations of people's pain and trauma have been dismissed. We didn't have the proper tools to understand exactly how the superhighway of the vagus nerve impacts virtually everything we do, including our ability to live comfortable, sociable lives, but we do now.

A way forward to balance and health

I've seen over and over that a better understanding of our biology – and specifically the vagus nerve – helps us to see our emotions from a different perspective. When we can participate in life with this more informed perspective, we can free ourselves from the emotional highs and lows that result from being stuck in the extremities of our internal thermostat's hot and cold states. We don't have to endure stretches of time feeling wound up, stressed out or unable to switch off. We don't need to fear sinking into a state of apathy, where we might feel unmotivated or hopeless for weeks or even months. With better vagal tone comes resilience and flexibility. We can bend and flow with the currents of life without getting stuck. Our inner monologue shifts from asking *What's wrong with me?* and *Why can't I handle this?* to saying *This is difficult, but I can cope. I'm going to be okay.*

You may not be in sync with your body's signals right now, but with more knowledge and the right tools, you can be. Your body wants all the same things you do: health, safety, balance and stability. In this book, I'll teach you to speak your body's language so you can converse with it and build a partnership that benefits you on so many levels. This two-way connection is the foundation of any successful nervous system work, and has the power to drastically improve physical and mental health, reduce stress and improve overall wellbeing. I've not only seen this happen time and time again, but I've experienced it myself in profound ways (see page 52).

Ironically, the fact that so many of us are suffering from physical and mental ailments with no clear root cause is a sign that our bodies are doing *exactly* what they were designed to do: something's not right, and they're letting us know. You'd think the first place we'd look for the source of our dysregulation would be our environment, but so often that isn't the case. It wasn't for me, and it isn't for many of my patients and students.

Every time we take on another new project at work despite being overloaded and experiencing frequent tension headaches, we'll likely find that going beyond our natural limits brings us to the point of exhaustion or even meltdown, forcing us to address our problems. But even then, rather than realising that the pressure at work is impacting our health, too many of us are more likely to turn the blame inward and tell ourselves things like, *I'm not coping as well as I should be*, or the classic: *I should be able to handle this.*

Our feelings of anxiety, shutdown, shame, anger or stress are canaries in the coalmine – they're the alarm warning us that we're bumping up against our neurobiological limits. When we're not fluent in the language of these messages, we don't understand what they're trying to tell us. All we know is that we don't like those feelings, so we look to squash them down as quickly as possible. The longer we ignore the messages our body is sending us, the harder they become to hear. But hearing those messages and then using that information to actively manage our emotional states is the first step on the path back to regulation.

The solution lies in learning how to fix that internal thermostat that was set too cold or too hot due to chronic and traumatic stress, and regulating the temperature so we can live comfortably again. Consider this book a user manual to your internal thermostat, which you can read once and use forever. Unlike other interventions for releasing stress and trauma, working with your nervous system is a practice that can be honed over time, and used anywhere at any time.

The reset we'll cover in this book doesn't involve multiple paid sessions, taking expensive pills, taking time off work, buying special equipment or changing your routine in any significant way. For the price of this book, I'll give you all the knowledge you need to regulate your nervous system. You'll be free to share that knowledge with anyone who's interested (legally, of course!), and by the final page, you'll have simple tools you can use anywhere to feel better at any moment. One of the most common questions people ask me about resetting their nervous system is 'What's the best exercise to regulate the nervous system?' The answer: there's no *one* exercise that does this. We each need particular tools and resources depending on where our nervous system thermostat is at that given moment.

When we build a relationship with our body and allow ourselves to move along with life's ebbs and flows, the challenges we face become more manageable, and we become more resilient. It's our job to understand the stories within us, especially when they refer to past traumas, and deploy the proper tools to respond. When we do, we equip ourselves to lead more fulfilling, confident and healthy lives, because we finally have the tools to address dysregulation at its source. Most importantly, we can see once and for all that the challenges we're facing are *not* all in our heads.

I hope that the things you discover in this book change the way you think about your life. The work we're about to do will reveal that the story told by your body's narrative is more significant than the story you tell with words. This is why nervous system work is one of the most transformative things you can do.

About this book

Before we continue on our journey, it's important to note that the strategies, suggestions and tools used in this book are based on my experiences and research as a former physiotherapist and now as a nervous system educator. They are not intended as a substitute for professional advice given by your healthcare or medical professionals.

The training in this book will teach you to recognise the things that cause you to perceive danger. With practice, you'll get better at recognising your body's warning signals and more skilled at guiding it gently back towards regulation. The biological systems you'll learn about in Part One will give you a much clearer understanding of your inner world and why you might be experiencing certain challenges. Resetting your nervous system requires your body and brain to relearn responses and shape themselves accordingly – so this isn't the type of book where you can just sit back and simply take information in. To experience the many benefits regulation brings, you'll have to do some work – but I promise it's worth it.

Throughout this book there will be opportunities for you to complete active and reflective exercises. These will be indicated by the symbols:

- active learning 🚴
- tuning in 🧘

In Part Two, you'll learn 21 simple but effective tools you can use in your most challenging moments to bring yourself back to your set point. I want you to actively engage with these tools and practise them regularly so they become second nature. When it comes to rewiring, there's no substitute for experiential learning. You can't learn to play the piano by only watching tutorials – you need to roll up your sleeves and play.

By the end of our time together, you'll be intimately acquainted with your own unique nervous system and have the exact tools you need to consciously bring it back to a calm, balanced state. Best of all, the power to do this will be in your hands, not the hands of specialists, doctors or external resources. By learning how to work *with* the one body you have, you'll be in a position to create positive change in your life, and become healthier and more resilient in the process.

The beauty of this approach is that we can start from where we are. There's no need to excavate past traumas, befriend shadow selves or share our darkest secrets before the real work of transformation can begin. That's not to say that type of work isn't useful or important – it is – but it isn't a prerequisite to starting a nervous system reset. And as you work through this reset, you'll start to feel different. You'll get to know yourself better, and become stronger and more resilient, which will put you in a better position to do the hard, emotional work when you're ready.

Important note

This reset may not be suitable for you if you know or suspect that your distress stems from unresolved PTSD that gets worse when you focus on your body. If this is the case for you, I recommend working one on one with a licensed psychiatrist who can support you through this work.

You can start improving your health today by using these tools to tune in to the messages your body is sending, and change the channel. Every time you do, you'll be strengthening your brain–body system and building the skills to identify your true needs and respond to them appropriately. Being able to regulate yourself in this way is truly transformative, and I suspect that's why you're here. You've been looking for answers and solutions for a long time. This time, I believe you've found them.

1

The nervous system states

Before we start to learn about the human nervous system and all its moving parts in greater depth, it's a good idea to take a bird's-eye view of the nervous system states we're all constantly moving between. We'll explore each of these states in greater detail as we work through the book, and you'll get to know what each of them *feels* and looks like for you – no two of us are wired exactly the same.

This is why working on your ability to tune in to your own bodily signals – what we call autonomic awareness – is such a big piece of this puzzle. When you can recognise which of the three primary states you're in – just right, too hot or too cold – and understand *why* you're in that state, you can identify the best way to start moving back towards that comfortable set point again. This is self-regulation.

Self-regulation

Self-regulation refers to your ability to manage your behaviours and helpfully express your emotions, wants and needs. It's been found to be positively linked with psychological wellbeing, including aspects of personal growth, life purpose and self-acceptance. It can be triggered by the need to maintain bodily 'homeostasis' or balance. Although self-regulation typically develops in childhood, the neuroplasticity of our brain and nervous systems allows it to be taught and learned throughout our life span.

Just-right state

Let's start with something comfortable – that internal set point where everything feels 'just right'. You don't need to understand the term yet, but we'll learn later that this is also known as the *ventral vagal state*. When we talk about being regulated, this is the state we're aiming to be in most of the time. Initially, that can feel like too much of a stretch, so the aim can simply be to begin to spend longer moments in this state. Even on your very best day, you'll move in and out of this state several times, because that's precisely what you're designed to do in order to meet the demands of various situations and tasks.

The window of tolerance

Although I've been referring to this state as *a* set point it isn't so much a single temperature as it is a range of temperatures within which we feel at our best, because our degree of nervous system activation matches what's happening in our environment. Psychologist Dan Siegel calls this range our *window of tolerance*, and it looks like this.

The window of tolerance

Too hot!
rage
anxiety
aggression
fear
panic

Stretch zone

Just right
coffee with a friend
going for a run
emails
Window of Tolerance
cooking dinner
waking up
reading
going on a date

Stretch zone

Too cold!
apathy
shutdown
burnout
sadness
hopelessness
loneliness
sleep

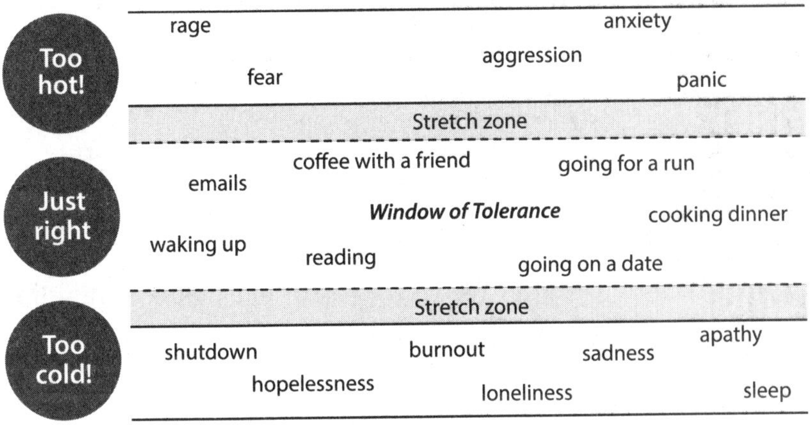

As you can see, the window of tolerance has an upper and lower boundary, and we experience fluctuations in energy and stress levels within the window. Your thermostat might turn up ever so slightly to get you energised for a date, or it might turn down a little during a quiet night in, but within these boundaries, you can tolerate your emotions and internal bodily sensations. For example, you might be excited or nervous about your date, but you can still think clearly, manage your moods and be in control of your emotions. In the golden zone of this just-right state, life feels pretty good, or at least perfectly manageable and within our control. We feel safe, calm and connected, and we can connect with others and the wider world around us.

At the upper and lower limits of this window are our *stretch zones* – where we can learn and grow in positive ways if we push ourselves (but not *too* much). When we're in one of our stretch zones, we can face challenges *without* crossing over into that hot or cold state. We may experience discomfort, but it shouldn't be so overwhelming that we can't cope. If you sign up for a marathon and start running for 30 minutes every other day, your stretch zone might look like adding 15 minutes to your run every week. Uncomfortable, yes, but necessary if you want to increase your stamina enough to eventually run for several hours.

As we saw earlier, stress isn't bad for us, we just need to be able to fully recover from it. We can learn to get better at building stress resilience and widening our window of tolerance rather than narrowing it and reducing our ability to cope by using a stress-reduction strategy. A stress-reduction strategy might include avoiding the things that are outside of our comfort zone or trying to control the behaviour of others.

How just right *feels* emotionally

You'll know you're in this state when you feel at home within yourself and at ease and able to express yourself well. Often, we're in this state when we're doing something we find engaging and motivating – this is what some people call *flow*. We feel present and communication is relatively easy. We access our social engagement system which is important for social bonding and attachment.

If our brain body system detects danger, this state can be thought of as our *first line of defence*, because it may involve engaging, negotiating and cooperating with another to end a threat. It may also involve yelling for help.

How just right *feels* in the body

- Heartbeat and breathing are even due to the cardiovascular regulation of the vagus nerve.

- Muscles are relaxed.
- Systems are working optimally.

Common thought patterns in the just-right state

- *I'm connected to my body.*
- *I'm connected to my environment.*
- *I'm connected to other people.*
- *I can cope with this.*
- *This feels challenging, but I can do it.*
- *I'm okay.*
- *I'm excited!*

What just right looks like

- Open or relaxed posture and movement.
- Good levels of eye contact.
- Smiling or other positive social cues.

How just right might sound in the voice

- Mid-range frequency – not too high, not too low.
- Calm, even pacing of speech.
- Friendly and curious tone.
- Controlled variation in rhythm and pitch.

Given how comfortable we are when we're in this state, you might assume that the goal of a nervous system reset is to learn how to stay in this state *all* the time – but it's not. After all, a nervous system that can't get angry is just as dysregulated as one that can't calm down. Our capacity to move in and out of all three states is what protects us from danger and allows us to mobilise our energy when we need to tap in to our strength and power. These are things that increase our agency, not to mention our likelihood of mastering a skill. It's perfectly healthy to move into fight-or-flight mode if there's a threat – in fact, it might save our life.

Rather than thinking of any of these states as good or bad, I invite you to see each of them not only as essential to living a rich life, but also to your survival. Your goal isn't to eliminate any of them, it's to understand *why* you're moving between them and then discern whether that move is justified based on the reality of your situation. Are you responding to *this* moment, or are you still responding to events from your past that feel similar? Learning how to shift into the appropriate state by influencing your unique patterns will help you live more optimally.

 Too hot state

This is our body's *second line of defence* also known as the *sympathetic state*, this provides the energy and primes our system to take action either by fighting or running away – in other words, the fight-or-flight response. When we shift into this state, we tend to do so very quickly because it's our 'emergency' state. In it, we're highly reactive and ready to respond to what our brain–body system deems to be life-or-death situations. Crossing the threshold from that just-right state into this much hotter state sets in motion a chain of powerful brain–body reactions. Because this is our do-or-die state, there's an emotional and physical intensity to it that makes it a very different experience from the other two.

How too hot *feels* emotionally

When we're in this state, we will notice that we become fearful, anxious and worried. We can feel strong urges to get up and do something, and it may feel impossible to sit still. Sometimes we can also feel constricted or trapped, along with the anger, rage and panic commonly associated with this state.

How too hot *feels* in the body

- Tension – often in the jaw, shoulders and spine.
- Stiffness in the neck muscles, especially around the larynx (voice box).
- Quicker heartbeat.
- The feeling of being on edge and unable to sit still.
- Dry mouth.
- Tight throat.
- Shallow, faster breathing (because we need more oxygen for fighting or fleeing).
- Shuddering or quivering.
- A surge of adrenaline (aka epinephrine) as neurochemicals are released.
- Heat or flushing through the chest or limbs (because blood flow is redirected from the digestive system towards the arms and legs to help them function optimally).
- Tightness in the hips or arms.
- Collectively these bodily signals could be grouped as anxiety, anger or rage.

Common thought patterns in the too hot state

When blood flow to the rational part of our brain slows down – as it does when we're in this state – there's more activity in what's known as our *survival brain*. This allows us to act swiftly from a place of instinct rather than thinking about things objectively or logically. The brain prioritises safety, efficiency and acting quickly, and we may lose sight of the big picture. The nervous system activation that occurs in this state will also cause us to hurry and go faster. Because of this switch, our thoughts might feel chaotic and uncontrollable, and be fear-based. We might tell ourselves:

- *Something bad is going to happen.*
- *I've got to do something now!*
- *Things will fall apart.*
- *I'm not going to succeed.*
- *I need to go faster.*

What too hot might look like

- Clenched jaw.
- Wide eyes.
- Tightly clenched fists.
- Fidgeting.
- Confrontational or evasive behaviour.

How too hot might sound in the voice

- Higher pitched (if panicked scared).
- Lower pitched (if angry or combative).
- Croaky.
- Faster speech.
- Verbal diarrhoea (the need to fill every moment of silence by talking).

Because this hotter state usually involves uncomfortable emotions and volatile or reactive behaviour, it's often demonised – but that's not entirely fair. This fight-or-flight state is essential to our survival, but when our brain–body system is detecting safety, this fiery, mobilising energy also helps us avoid exhaustion, apathy, forgetfulness, fogginess and extreme procrastination. It gives us strength and focus. Burnout, for example, an increasingly common condition these days, can be seen as a depletion of that mobilising energy combined with low vagal tone.

In truth, challenges (or what we call stressors) can bring lots of positive adaptations *provided* we get to recover from these experiences. As we learned earlier, this process is known as allostasis, meaning we have the innate capacity to meet demands and recover from them. An activated state may trigger immune cells to travel to a part of the body where a pathogen (a microorganism that causes disease) has been detected. It might also cause the brain to secrete the stress hormone cortisol and our muscles to release stored glucose in response. This 'emergency' glucose gives our brain extra energy, and the circulating cortisol improves memory about the current situation. This promotes learning and also ensures we're less likely to make the same mistake in the future. As our physical and emotional demands change throughout the day, our blood pressure rises and falls to help us focus or perform a difficult task.

It's only when stress is too overwhelming or repeated too many times that the wear and tear from being in this hotter state starts to become evident. Neurons (brain cells) in our survival brain might make new connections that make us more prone to fear and hypersensitive to threat. Hormones might dysregulate our immune function, making us more susceptible to illness or prone to inflammation. This is why we often get sick following long periods of stress. Constantly elevated blood pressure might also allow atherosclerotic plaques to develop in our arteries (aka hardening of the arteries), making us even more prone to elevated blood pressure.

Hyperawareness of bodily signals

If anxiety is part of your hot state, you may become overly attentive to internal signals coming from your body, but you may not be able read them accurately. For example, your brain might misread a small fluctuation in your heart rate as a much bigger danger signal than it actually is, causing you to become even more anxious. This occurs because chronic and traumatic stress can increase the connectivity between the part of the brain that processes messages from the nervous system and the regions of the brain that govern fear. This can amplify our sense of panic, and these sensations can ultimately become overwhelming.

❄ Too cold state

This is our *third line of defence* also known as the *dorsal vagal state*, and unlike the hot state, which is one of activation, the cold state is one of energy conservation. This immobilisation is usually the critical point in a life-threatening traumatic event and we either freeze or shutdown and collapse.

In addition to collapse and immobility, the cold state also impacts communication, so that it becomes almost impossible to speak up for ourselves. Some studies have indicated that one of the primary areas of the brain for expression, known as the Broca's area, goes offline when there are very high levels of activity in our fear circuitry. This is why talking about what's happening in this state is not helpful. Instead, we need to connect with our body.

Dissociation

People commonly describe feeling disconnected or 'cut off' from their body when stuck in the too cold state. This sensation is very real, because when we move into this state, our body releases endorphins to increase our pain tolerance, while causing us to feel disconnected from our environment and also other people. This is the body's way of protecting us on a psychological level, and if you've ever been in a state of shock following an accident or other traumatic event, you'll have a good idea how this feels.

The numbness this disconnection creates is known as dissociation or functional 'disappearing'. It's the equivalent of pulling the hand brake in a car and coming to a complete stop. This happens because when we experience something traumatic, it's less distressing for us to not feel events that are happening in terms of pain and emotions. In the short term this hand brake helps us to cope, but in the long term, dissociation has negative effects on the body and the neurological system.

In one study of adults with depression, the ability to make decisions based on bodily signals was reduced. When we're not well connected to our body and its sensations, it can cause emotional numbness – an overall sense that we can't feel anything at all. When our networks block out our bodily sensations to 'protect us', that two-way connectivity between the brain and the body via the vagus nerve can also be dampened, and so may our ability to maintain homeostasis of our systems. This can be the root cause of some chronic health conditions, including lower back pain, persistent pain, IBS, anxiety and depression.

When we can only recognise heightened states, we can't actively take care of our emotions. For example, we might not notice that we're getting angry until it escalates to rage. This robs us of the opportunity to pivot out of that growing anger to become grounded and calm, because we've already shifted into anger, panic, freeze or survival mode.

When we're in this cold state we might freeze – just like a deer in the headlights of an oncoming car. When people wonder why someone in danger didn't just get out of there or fight back, the answer is usually because that person went into a state of freeze or shutdown in which taking action was physically impossible. Unfortunately, while the 'fight' response is often praised in our society when someone is facing a traumatic experience, a freeze or immobilisation response is judged harshly due to a lack of understanding of how the nervous system works when we face a life-threatening situation. This can lead to feelings of shame in the person who froze, which is unfair because in the moment, we can't always control how our brain–body system reacts to sudden and overwhelming danger.

If our brain-body system detects safety then this is the state where sleep, deep relaxation and recovery functions for our organs takes place.

How too cold *feels* emotionally

- Lack of safety.
- Hopelessness.
- Depression.
- Exhaustion.
- Dulled emotions.
- Disconnection from the body and environment.
- Like being alone in a dark room.
- A lack of belonging (shame).

How too cold *feels* in the body

- A rapid reduction of heart rate (known as bradycardia) and breathing rate.
- A drop in energy.
- Sluggish digestion.
- Cold hands and feet (since blood moves to the centre of the body).
- Numbness.
- Fogginess.

Common thought patterns in the too cold state

- *Everything is hopeless.*
- *There's nothing I can do.*
- *I'm too tired to try.*
- *Nothing I do will ever be good enough.*
- *What do I have to offer?*

What too cold looks like

- Slumped, rounded shoulders.

- Sunken chest.
- Lack of eye contact.
- Lack of interest.
- Dropped head.
- Blank face (collapse).
- Wide eyes (in a freeze state).
- Averted gaze (shame).

How too cold might sound in the voice

- Inability to speak.
- Monotone.
- Lower pitch.
- Quieter volume.
- Slower speech.
- Mumbling.

Nervous System State	Brain–Body System Detects Threat	Brain–Body System Detects Safety
Just right Ventral Vagal	**First line of defence** Looking around for danger and people to recruit to help. Talking, negotiating and cooperating with others until the threat is over.	**Safe and social** Bonding and attachment. Emotions feeling manageable.
Too hot Sympathetic	**Second line of defence** Mobilising energy for fight or flight.	Mobilising energy to face challenges and meet demands. (See Play on page 55.)
Too cold Dorsal Vagal	**Third line of defence** Immobilising energy, and freezing or shutdown.	Sleep, deep relaxation and recovery functions for organs and systems. (See Stillness on page 56.)

One party, different states

Let's take a look at how people in their too hot or too cold states might react to the stress of attending a party.

Flight

Tonight's party has been on Laura's mind ever since her co-worker invited her a few weeks ago. She hasn't been to a party since moving to this city six months ago – she isn't sure she even remembers how to socialise. In bed at night, Laura's been having racing thoughts about how this party will go. She worries that she'll be awkward and that people will think she's weird. What will she do if someone makes fun of her? What if she says the wrong thing?

On her way there, Laura feels hypervigilant and on edge. Her palms are sweaty and her heart races. After saying a quick hi to the host, she spends the next 20 minutes standing near the front door with her arms tightly folded across her chest. While making small talk with colleagues from work, she thinks *I'm talking so fast!* Although she knows some of them fairly well, for some reason she only feels comfortable talking about surface-level topics like the weather or TV shows.

Laura's inability to be vulnerable in any way is one of the many symptoms of her hotter activated state. Physically, her fast breathing, clammy palms and tense shoulders are signalling back to her brain that she's in danger, and her brain is creating thoughts to support this (e.g. *I'm talking so fast!*). This feedback loop between her brain and body are keeping her in flight mode and preventing her from shifting into a cooler state, where she'd be able to relax and connect with her friends at the party.

Fight

Like Laura, Renee has been dreading tonight. Even though she's friends with the host and was pleased to be invited, Renee's past experiences of being bullied have recently been triggered with ongoing conflict at work that has resulted in insomnia, and so she has been unconsciously preparing to face a similar type of rejection at the party.

After handing her friend a gift, Renee grabs a drink and unknowingly adopts a closed and defensive posture in a corner of the kitchen. She stands with her back against a wall, gripping the strap of her purse in her fist. Her muscles are tense, and her eyes scan the room, even as she chats to a few people she knows. At times she even scowls, though she doesn't realise she's doing it. 'She's got that look on her face,' one of her friends says. So they steer clear, assuming she's in a bad mood. Renee notices that her friends have avoided her and this sends a surge of heat through her chest and arms and she feels her hands reflexively move into fists. To those who don't know her, she appears unfriendly – even threatening.

When a friend calls her over to include her in a conversation, Renee tries to relax and join in with the jokey banter. But when she mistakenly thinks a harmless joke is directed at her, she reacts badly and the woman who made the joke quickly excuses herself from the group. Though the others continue to talk, Renee's over-reaction makes them less inclined to interact with her, increasing her feelings of isolation.

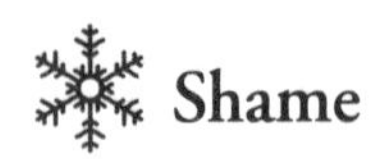

Shame

Samin's confidence took a big hit when her long-term partner broke up with her. Shortly after this, she was forced to give up the city apartment they'd shared and move in with her parents to save money. These big life changes left her incredibly deflated, and she feels deep shame about losing her relationship *and* the city lifestyle she loved in such a short time. The idea of ever being able to afford a place of her own and meeting someone great again seems hopeless.

Since moving back in with her parents, Samin has slipped out of her regular routine. Evening walks around the park and cooking herself healthy meals for the week have been replaced with nights in front of the TV with her parents and overly generous helpings of her mother's cooking. She's put on some weight and is convinced that the people at the party tonight will see her and think, *Wow, Samin's let herself go since her breakup!*

At the party, she catches up with a couple she knows. They've just bought their first house and are telling her about their plans for extending their kitchen. Samin smiles and nods along, but she's deflated on the inside and only half-listening. All she can think is, *God, I hope they don't ask where I'm living.* She's terrified they'll judge her for moving home. The more they talk, the more she feels that her life has moved backwards, not forwards. *Why did I even come here tonight?* she thinks.

Samin's energy is noticeably flat, and before long the couple shift their attention to the other people sitting nearby. Samin barely notices. She slumps back in the chair and sips her drink. She feels like she's hardly in the room, let alone part of the group. Like Laura and Renee, Samin's physical posture is influencing her thoughts, and that constant feedback loop is reinforcing her belief that she's not good enough and amplifying her feelings of shame.

*

In the same way a wild antelope returns to grazing with its herd after outrunning a lion, we have the ability to leap into frenzied action and return to a calmer state once a threat has passed – but *only* if we have a well-regulated nervous system and our prior experiences shape how this process takes place. Theoretically, all three of our party guests have the innate ability to shift back to a calmer, more collected baseline in the safe and friendly environment of the party. But since all three remained in their agitated or hopeless states even after other guests tried connecting with them, they might be stuck outside of their window of tolerance.

How do we get stuck in these states?

As mentioned earlier, a well-regulated nervous system is one that can shift in and out of the three states as needed via allostasis and return to its optimal set point. But if life is stressful for long enough and we don't know how to bring ourselves back to that just-right state, we run the risk of staying stuck at a non-optimal temperature, which causes us to suffer both mentally and physically. Chronic or traumatic stress can lead to three possible patterns of nervous system dysregulation:

1. We get stuck in the hot state.
2. We get stuck in the cold state.
3. We oscillate between the two extremes.

Tom and Sophia's story: Stuck in opposite states

For most of us, getting stuck in one of these states is not something we see coming, as was the case for Tom and Sophia, a married couple in their late twenties. When Tom's mother, Betty, was diagnosed with a particularly aggressive terminal cancer, he and Sophia volunteered to become her primary carers. Neither of them had any experience of caring for someone with a terminal illness, or been close to death before, but they were committed to supporting Betty in any way they could.

The year they spent caring for Betty affected each of them in profound but very different ways. As their story illustrates, which pattern we fall into during times of stress is unpredictable, because how stress manifests for each of us looks different.

 Stuck in the hot state

When our thermostat gets turned up to hot, also known as the state of hyperarousal, our body responds quickly and with intensity. This is an asset in the heat of the moment, but far less beneficial if we get stuck there. When we lose the ability to relax or switch off (as we do when we're in survival mode), we may get startled easily and feel prolonged hyper vigilance, anxiety, irritation and anger. The heightened emotions that often accompany this state can also make it easy for us to overreact to situations. We may storm off, say things we don't mean, blame others unfairly, start arguments or just generally be far spikier and more reactive than we would be in our regulated state.

In order to cope, you might find yourself *over*doing certain things in an effort to bring yourself back into regulation. You might exercise too much, thinking it will get rid of your nervous energy, overwork or set unreasonable expectations for yourself so you can feel more in control, and then rely on caffeine, sugar and stimulants to keep you going. The hormones that flood our body in those do-or-die moments overstay their welcome, and the changes to our immune system make us prone to things like gastrointestinal problems, insomnia and aches and pains.

As long as the system that governs this hot state is running the show, the biological functions that contribute to our long-term survival will continue to be set aside in order to free up all available physical resources for the immediate effort of survival. If this continues for long periods, essential functions relating to digestion and our immune response will remain on the back burner because the body is sending the brain the physiological message that we're fighting for our lives. In such a scenario, breaking down lunch is less important than keeping the heart rate elevated. It also means that vital processes such as cellular repair or our clean-up systems aren't working at their best, magnifying whatever wear and tear is occurring, and opening the door for new illnesses to emerge.

When this state persists for a long time, it can lead to allostatic load building up. For example, blood pressure rises in the face of danger, but when it rises repeatedly – as it can if someone has a stressful work situation – those blood pressure changes become chronic and can result in our nervous system set point being raised to a higher temperature.

Sophia: Stuck in the hot state

While caring for Betty, Sophia found herself becoming increasingly antsy and unsettled. Having to call the ambulance a few times when Betty was struggling to breathe increased her anxiety, and before long her mind was dominated by fear. She worried that she'd accidentally give Betty the wrong dose of medicine, or cause an infection by not sterilising something properly.

When Betty passed away, both Sophia and Tom were at her

bedside. Though her death was relatively peaceful, the experience shocked them deeply. Following Betty's death, Sophia became hypervigilant – checking the street five or six times before crossing, and worrying about the health consequences of things she'd previously thought nothing of. She checked food labels obsessively, stopped using the microwave, and eventually even stopped using her mobile phone and laptop – worried that radiation from these devices might cause cancer.

The year of intense stress and heartache had taken a heavy toll on Sophia, and though she hadn't battled cancer herself, the proximity to such a frightening situation not only pulled her into an overheated state, but caused her to remain stuck there. Physically, she began suffering from regular tension headaches and digestive problems. Her baseline set point had been well and truly shifted, and this once carefree young woman saw herself in a very different light than she had just one year earlier. When asked to describe herself, she was prone to say things like:

- 'I'm just a worry wart, that's all.'
- 'I've always been an anxious person, so I'm sure that's what it is.'
- 'I'll just start taking the nutrient labels off of everything so I don't even think to look.'
- 'I'll get over it; I just need to stop being a wimp.'

Spending too long in this hot state resulted in Sophia accidentally creating a new set point for herself – one she couldn't thrive in. Being stuck in this state was, of course, not something Sophia was choosing. It happened outside of her conscious awareness, when her nervous system was under too much stress and she had no period of recovery. It's normal for all of us to have anxious tendencies once in a while, but becoming chronically anxious to the point that we have over-the-top reactions to non-threatening events is an indication that our thermostat has reset itself at a hotter set point. Sophia's new set point was quite a bit higher than her original one, which was why she was operating from a baseline of anxiety almost all the time.

❄ Stuck in a cold state

In this state, we're unlikely to be able to muster up enough energy to meet life's demands, so when faced with stressors, we *under*cope. If we spend too long in this state, we might feel foggy and numb, experience depression, forgetfulness and clumsiness, and have low libido. We may also feel sluggish even after getting plenty of sleep. If we stay stuck in this state of hypoarousal for long enough, we may even feel tired all the time.

When we're in this state, we can feel powerless, hopeless and even depressed. That's why it's so easy to find yourself glued to the couch and binge-watching TV after facing something challenging that pulls you out of your comfort zone. If you remain in this chronic state of hypoarousal, you might find yourself procrastinating and avoiding things you know you should do. You might start to isolate yourself from people and even stop leaving the house as much.

Tom: Stuck in the cold state

Despite living through the same experience as Sophia, Tom's nervous system reacted very differently. In the weeks after his mother's death, Tom took time off work and couldn't get out of bed. Despite sleeping for much of the day, he felt constantly exhausted and took very little interest or joy in hobbies he once loved. Once he got back to work, moving through the day often felt painful and disorienting. At times, he noticed that he felt completely disconnected from himself and the world. He felt foggy, numb and forgetful.

He went from being someone who enjoyed his work and was often up for a night out with his friends, to feeling utterly uninterested. So much so that he couldn't seem to start or finish projects or return texts and calls when friends reached out. He couldn't escape feelings of gloom and hopelessness, and had no idea how to make himself feel better.

After months of missing work deadlines and avoiding friends, he no longer liked or understood the person he'd become. He started saying things like:

- 'I'm just a lazy person.'
- 'I'm an antisocial person.'
- 'I'm going to give myself shorter deadlines so I feel pressure to finish my work.'
- 'I'm going to make myself go to the party on Saturday. I'll have a coffee beforehand to get myself energised.'
- 'I've lost my mojo. I've lost my motivation.'

Oscillating between two extremes

Sometimes, instead of being stuck in one state, we get stuck swinging between states, and how that looks is different for each of us. If you find yourself in this state, you may experience several days or even weeks in that hotter state – like the 'on' button is jammed or you're wired or you've drunk too much coffee and you feel like you can't slow down – only to crash with fatigue, pain, illness or a tension headache. You might alternate between periods of insomnia and excessive sleep. For some people, extreme behaviour can be an indication that they're stuck in this state, as it's often a hallmark of someone who is masking, suppressing, denying, self-medicating or coping with extreme dysregulation the best they know how. As with the example of Tom and Sophia, the catalyst for getting stuck in this pattern is rarely one we see coming and it's certainly not something we choose to do.

My own story: Swinging from hot to cold and back again

At university, I was taught how important it is to make my work patient-centred. I still take great care not to centre myself as I support people through their transformation towards nervous system regulation. In this context, however, sharing some of what I've experienced will highlight how easy it is for anyone to slip into this dysregulated state. Several years ago, I was pushing myself hard at the physiotherapy practice I'd started. I was juggling a full caseload of patients while also managing the many day-to-day administrative demands of a busy practice. There were never enough hours in the day, and looking back on that time now, it's clear to me that I spent most of those days in a too hot state – running on the mobilising energy of my dysregulated nervous system, while feeling pulled in all directions.

My body was sending me signals, of course, but I became good at blocking those out and pushing through. Eventually, I pushed myself straight into burnout, and when I started to experience digestive issues for the first time in my life, I assumed it was because I was eating too many meals on the run. It didn't occur to me that it could be linked to the constant pressure of work.

When my brother, Sam, died, I was flung without warning into the hardest phase of my life. Burnout and stress were compounded by a deep, inescapable grief, and I spent the next year swinging wildly between my hot and cold states. It was only when I began searching for a way back to myself that I discovered nervous system regulation, which turned out to be the path back to health and stability for me. Finding this work was like a lightbulb moment and, to be honest, when I learned about the way my nervous system was working it felt like coming home. I no longer felt helpless and out of control.

Many people who take my nervous system reset course do so after experiencing the sudden loss of a child or loved one. The shock of death throws us out of our current state, and if we're already facing other stresses when this happens, the effects can be significant and long-lasting – despite the saying, time *doesn't* heal all wounds. It could also occur after years of experiencing anxiety and depression following a difficult childhood. Or it could come after months or years of living under traumatic stress. That doesn't mean, however, we can't return to balance. I hope my story illustrates how much progress can be made by harnessing the body's inbuilt capabilities to cope, and most importantly, recalibrate. Although life will never be the same after some painful experiences, our body can find its way back to regulation again so that we can feel at home inside ourselves. I still miss Sam and feel sadness that he's no longer here, but I'm not dysregulated by his loss.

Dysregulation strikes us all differently

Tom and Sophia illustrate how differently dysregulation can show up in response to the same stimulus. Neither of them chose to respond to Betty's death the way they did – their life experiences and bodily responses guided them in two different directions. Frequently, in a situation where both members of a couple are dysregulated, they might start to shift blame and shame onto one another – and themselves – even unintentionally. If we're not aware of having a just-right state in the first place, we're unlikely to have the resources or knowledge to bring us back to our calmer, more connected old self. Instead, we get stuck, shrinking our window of tolerance and convincing ourselves that we have to just get over it and power through, regardless of how we're feeling.

My life was so changed by my experience of learning to regulate my nervous system that I left a 13-year career as a physiotherapist to dedicate myself to spreading the message that it *is* absolutely possible to restore wellness by returning our nervous system to a healthy set point. One of the greatest benefits of learning to partner with our body is that we no longer get stuck in one of these states for prolonged periods, thus, saving ourselves from so much unnecessary suffering. Building vagal tone and working with our body also widens our window of tolerance, making it easier for us to maintain equilibrium and stay within our just-right state, even while facing tough challenges.

The secondary states

The three nervous system states we've just explored aren't the only ones we move in and out of. There are three more states – our secondary or 'blended' states – and they're equally important to our wellbeing. At any given point of the day, we are in one of the primary or blended states.

If we picture the three primary states as primary colours, we can imagine how, when mixed in different combinations, they'd create different shades, with unique tones and moods:

- too hot – red
- just right – yellow
- too cold – blue.

Play

When the yellow of our just-right state is mixed with a touch of mobilising red, this creates the orange of play – the state in which we feel energised and excited, but also safe and social. For example, this could be going to a comedy show with a friend, singing karaoke, dancing, playing a game with children or skating with a partner. Ideally it's reciprocal, and you feel both mobilised and connected to another person.

Experiencing awe, motivation, passion or inspiration also leads to this state. We might shift into it when we hike to the top of a ridge and encounter a breathtaking view, or when we take in the beauty of a foreign city. Many of us also experience this state when we participate in something bigger than ourselves, such as creating a collectively beautiful sound as a choir or chanting with the crowd in a sports stadium. We can also enter this play state when speaking or teaching about a topic we love and are passionate about.

Peak performance may arise from the blend of these two states, such as an athlete or a leader making decisions in a high-pressured situation.

Moving into our play state is a way to exercise our nervous system to be more flexible, adaptable and resilient when we experience the mobilising energy of our sympathetic nervous system.

Your experience of being in the play state will be unique – not only to you, but also depending on the experience that causes the shift. How you feel on a night out with your closest friends, for example, is unlikely to mirror the emotions and thoughts you have while swimming in a lake – although you're likely to be in the play state for both experiences.

You can download a free play worksheet at www.jessicamaguire.com/play.

Stillness

Like a rolling green meadow, the state of stillness is created when we blend the calm yellow energy of our window of tolerance with the blue of our cold state. Stillness is a highly restorative state, and the one we might shift into when we're doing something introspective and quiet – a deep meditation, perhaps, or lying on our mat at the end of a yoga class. Sharing an intimate moment with another person, as a mother does when she's breastfeeding, can also put us in this state. Unsurprisingly, it's also the state we're in when we fall asleep.

Freeze

Freeze is the state we shift into when threatened, and it's a blend of the two extreme states. When a dab of fight-or-flight red energy is mixed with a blob of immobilising blue, we feel both of those energies, though the purple of collapse or shutdown is the dominant energy. We might feel activation, heat and energy through our body, but at the same time our feet might feel as though they're stuck in cement. Our breath might freeze as well, and we might notice tightness in the muscles between our ribs.

A shift into the freeze state can occur when we feel activated and angry but also paralysed and unable to take action, such as in a confrontation or conflict when we know we need to be brave and stand up for ourselves.

Unlike play and stillness, which are enjoyable, rejuvenating and restorative, freeze isn't a particularly pleasant state to be in. It is, however, a part of life. This immobilisation is designed to protect us. It is also, unfortunately, poorly understood by our society, which often can't understand why someone doesn't 'just fight back'. This lack of nervous system understanding can create more shame for a trauma victim. Thankfully, the tools you'll learn for shifting out of that too cold state can also help to get you out of this freeze state. You'll find those in Part Two of this book.

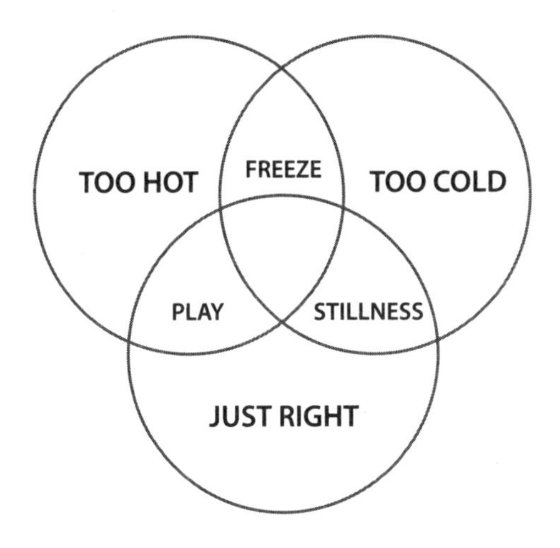

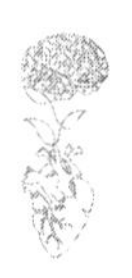

Each colour on this palette is beautiful and unique, but if we can only paint with a few of them, the result may feel flat and cartoonish. The freedom to switch between all of the colours and blend them together to match the changing light is what brings richness, dimension and depth. The ability to do this without getting 'stuck' in one particular state is what makes us flexible and adaptable. This is how we paint a picture that reflects the reality of our external world.

Two other blended states include appeasement and fawn, and these relate to relational experiences where there is abuse or life-threat, and where we may try to help our perpetrator feel calm.

Appeasement is considered a blend of all three states – this is where we become a 'super regulator' for someone who is very threatening. We would use our social engagement system of our just-right state to be a co-regulator for another person, particularly someone who has a much higher position of power than us, or it's a life-threatening situation. There would still be a blob of the too hot or sympathetic energy that would have us on guard, and we would likely be dissociated from our sense of self because of the too cold or dorsal vagal energy. It involves all three states and acts like a 'super' social engagement system that someone takes on and sends cues of regulation, or enmeshes with the person who is life-threatening.

Fawn is a blended state that *doesn't* include the ventral vagal state. There's the sympathetic activation which makes us hyper-vigilant and we'll be on the lookout for the other person's changes in cues, behaviours, actions. And then there's the dorsal vagal energy, that results in us dissociating from our own feelings, our values and our own agency. We submit to who it is that holds power or is abusive. We'll submit that power or the decision to the other person. It may feel as though our sense of self disappears or we're invisible. That 'hiding' comes from dorsal vagal energy.

Both appeasement and fawn are survival strategies; our body's way of trying to keep us safe when there's life-threat – this is not the same as people pleasing.

By the end of this book, you will have learned many tools and resources that work best for your unique system. To reset your nervous system, you will need to make these resources part of your daily practices. Incorporating regulating practices into your daily routine couldn't be easier, and as you start mapping out how this will look for you, I invite you to take a moment and reflect on why you're doing this.

Read the questions below and write down your responses in a notebook or journal you can come back to, and pop a reminder in your calendar to revisit these answers in three months, six months or next year – or all three. They'll show you just how incredible your brain–body system is, and how quickly it can help you improve your life and realise your goals. You might see this phenomenon expressed as 'salience matters'. In other words, to achieve real change, your goal must be something that is important to you.

- What's your intention with resetting your nervous system thermostat?
- Is it to be more present and free to enjoy life?
- Is it to improve the health of your relationships?
- Is it to flourish, thrive and reach your potential?
- Spend some time reflecting on and identifying what matters most to you and write down your goals for your nervous system reset.

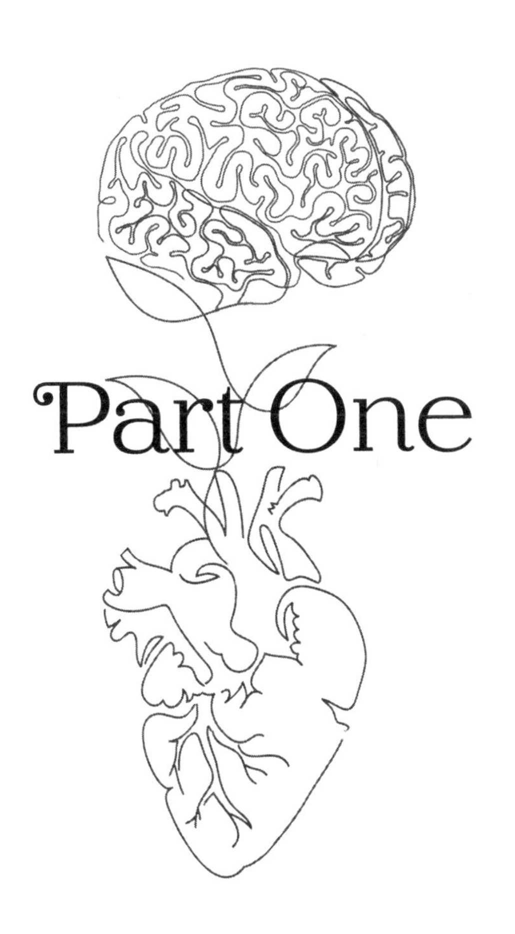

Part One

Foundation and framework

A nervous system primer

Since we can't reset what we don't understand, increasing our knowledge about the nervous system is the best place to start. This foundation will provide a clear framework on which you can hang the tools you'll be learning in Part Two. Over the next few chapters, we'll explore how our nervous system gathers information, what the various systems within this large network look like and how they function. By the end, you'll have so much more insight into the incredible biological machinery at your disposal. You'll also have a much better understanding of why it plays such a big role in how well (or unwell) you feel.

Don't sweat the science

I know the foundational science presented in this book can get a little complex – it's neuroscience! – but I encourage you to embrace the complexities.

The science is included here to help show you how intricate the brain–body system is, and how interconnected our nervous system is with other vital body systems, such as the immune, endocrine and digestive. This helps us really see how things like traumatic stress may make you more likely to develop a gut disorder and how you can influence this.

This is where nervous system work is both an art and a science.

But importantly, you don't have to fully grasp all the technical intricacies and science for this reset to work for you. You can, of course, revisit some of the more technical sections as your understanding of the nervous system grows.

If you're reading this book because you know or suspect that your nervous system is dysregulated, you may be planning to skip these next chapters and look for the solution to your specific challenge or problem. Believe me, I understand that impulse. Please trust me, though. It would be a mistake to skip these foundational chapters, because they contain many of the explanations you've been searching for.

Besides, if you've been looking for answers for a long time, surely there's nothing more interesting than the inner workings of a system that's been keeping you alive since birth. Your nervous system has been shaping your experience of life at the most foundational level since your mother's pregnancy, and will continue to do so for the rest of your days. Consider the time you spend reading the next five chapters as an investment in your health and a gift to your future self.

I've taught thousands of people to work with their nervous system, and the questions I hear most frequently are 'What can I do to fix my insomnia/IBS/anxiety?' and 'What's the best exercise to build vagal tone?' They want me to point them to one specific exercise or course module that will finally solve this problem for them, quickly. I tell them the same thing I'm about to tell you: the first thing we must do when tackling any type of nervous system dysregulation is shift our mind in one major way.

We have to learn to look beyond the health or emotional difficulty we're experiencing and identify the nervous system state that's causing it.

Once we've done that, our priority is bringing ourselves back into a regulated state and progressing from there.

In the image of the iceberg on page 12 we can see that trying to tackle dysregulation by focusing on its individual symptoms is like playing whac-a-mole. If we don't address the situations causing our underlying dysregulation, we stay stuck outside our window of tolerance, unable to make meaningful progress. Sure, we might be able to smack down one or two symptoms, but for how long? Another will pop up soon enough, and that's no way to live. It keeps us trapped in a cycle of reacting to problems rather than preventing them from occurring in the first place.

That's why this nervous system reset starts with lifting the lid on our neurobiology. This goes beyond cognitively knowing something. You need to recognise what's happening in your body's signals and its narrative. Together, we're going to take a good look at the machinery at work under the surface. Once you understand how the pieces fit together, you'll have a radically different perspective on your wellbeing. You'll get better at identifying the mechanisms propelling each of those 'moles' to the surface, and you'll become skilled at switching them off at their source.

In the context of your nervous system, this involves taking active steps to regulate your state. You'll improve your health and quality of life in the process, and even lower your risk of future illnesses. This sounds like a grand promise, I know, but scientific research, especially into allostatic load – cumulative wear and tear on the body that shifts our set point – has linked chronic stress to serious illness. As we've discovered, this includes persistent pain, digestive issues, sleep disorders and inflammation.

The body can't use words to recall or communicate its experiences, so it does this through movement – by tightening, bracing, collapsing, withdrawing, freezing or holding. Sensations, breathing patterns and heartbeat are other ways it tries to tell us how it's doing. Learning the language of this brain–body system is one of the most powerful ways I know to adapt to life's changes in a healthy, regulated way. Research conducted over the past two decades has demonstrated that working with the body's signals can help shift us back towards regulation following chronic and traumatic stress.

Though the details behind these communication pathways can often get a bit complex and science-y, it's important to understand that your nervous system can and will change throughout your life. In this very moment it's being shaped by the things you're experiencing and thinking, as well as the environment you're in and the relationships you have. These things influence the activity and also the structure of the brain. In turn, that reshaping can trigger physical changes in other important systems – namely the endocrine system (which is responsible for hormone release) and the immune system.

It can feel intimidating to learn that the brain–body system is constantly moulding itself in response to every good and bad experience we have, but I assure that you this is actually great news. It means we can play an active role in that shaping process, too, via bioplasticity – a concept we'll explore and put to use in Part Two. In the same way we can shape our muscles at the gym, we can sculpt our brain–body system in order to live a more regulated, centred life – one with less emotional distress and physical discomfort.

If the information in this part of the book feels overwhelming at any point, slow down. Remind yourself why it's important and take time to connect the biology you're reading about with the incredible things going on inside your body right now. As you read these very words your heart is pumping, your lungs are breathing and your nervous system is firing messages to and from your brain at an incomprehensible speed. I'm going to help you tap in to these messages, interpret what they're telling you and influence what they're saying.

My life changed for the better after I learned I had the power to do this, and I know yours will too.

2

Our four fact-finding networks

At the most simplistic level, our nervous system is a series of networks gathering and sending information. Like a global news corporation headquartered in a major city, it manages four major networks, each with its own foreign correspondents working 24/7 to collect updates for head office (the brain). Most of the information sent to head office is good intel collected from accurate sources, but some of it – especially information regarding danger – is less reliable and can be harder to translate. If head office doesn't fact check this info or gather more intel to put it in context, it might run a story that isn't true or send orders to the networks that aren't appropriate to the unfolding situation. Unfortunately, this happens more often than we'd like.

By understanding how the four major networks are connected to each other and to the brain, and how they affect each other and our brain–body system, we can learn to better regulate ourselves. Many of us learn about our 'five senses' from an early age, but what most of us aren't taught is that those are just one of our *four* fact-finding systems. Three of them gather information from *inside* our bodies and it's this information that tells our brain how we're doing so it can maintain that optimal just-right state of homeostasis. Each system gathers a different type of information, but they share the same purpose: to warn us of danger and keep us safe.

Network 1: The exteroceptive system (the five senses)

The five exteroceptive senses – from the Latin *exterus* meaning 'exterior' and the English 'perception' – are the most obvious of our four fact-finding systems, as they involve visible organs that we use consciously as well as subconsciously to gather information from the environment *outside* our body through:

1. touch
2. taste
3. sight
4. sound
5. smell.

Sensory cells called exteroceptors send input from our tongue, skin, eyes, ears and nose to the brain. There, information is filtered, processed and integrated so the brain can decide how to respond – this is called exteroception. If our mum always made brownies for the annual family reunion, then – as an adult – the smell of chocolate is likely to evoke happy feelings in us. Conversely, if we lived through a house fire in our childhood, the smell of smoke or sight of a fire engine might trigger feelings of fear or panic.

This exteroceptive system is also responsible for gathering information about our social world – primarily about our environment and how the people within it are reacting to us. If we're floating on our back in a calm ocean and looking at the sky, the feeling of the water lapping against our skin and the sight of the clouds above will likely make us feel relaxed. If, however, we're standing on the shore with wind whipping against our face, and we can hardly hear the person next to us and can see that they look scared and are shouting, the information we're gathering from our exteroceptive network will make us feel decidedly uneasy, even fearful.

Network 2: The proprioceptive system (the sixth sense)

Contrary to the premise of a certain 1990s movie, our sixth sense has nothing to do with seeing dead people – at least not in the context of biology. It's the system that makes us aware of our body's location at any given moment, including when we're in motion, named for the Latin *proprius*, meaning 'one's own' and the English 'perception'. Receptors in joints, muscles and tendons all over our body send signals to our brain, letting it know where certain body parts are. It's how we can close our eyes and touch our nose, or step off a curb without needing to look down.

We start forming a brain map of our body through touch and movement in the womb, and more detail is added to this map as we start to grab, kick, touch, crawl, walk and run. This sixth sense is how we can learn physical movements to the point they become automatic – as with surfing or dancing. With enough practice, this 'muscle memory' means we'll intuitively know where to position our feet and how to move our legs and arms automatically to perform the desired movement while maintaining balance. And speaking of balance . . .

Network 3: The vestibular system (the seventh sense)

The vestibular system is located in our inner ear, and the information it gathers tells our brain about the position of our head in space. This helps us coordinate eye movements, adjust our posture and maintain our balance. Like our other systems, it develops in infancy through changes in position, such as being rocked or gently swung, and evolves through movements such as rolling, crawling, walking and running.

This vestibular system is what allows us to keep our balance and maintain a comfortable relationship with gravity. It's at work any time we practise a downward dog in yoga, bounce on a therapy ball or spin around a dance floor. It helps us maintain balance while integrating information coming from our proprioceptive and exteroceptive systems.

We rarely engage this seventh sense consciously, but if you're particularly attuned to it, you might be the type of air passenger who can sense turns and changes in altitude on a plane without having to look out of a window. When this system isn't functioning as it should, we might experience vertigo, dizziness or loss of balance. Learning how to work with this system is essential if we want to become adept at moving into a calm, regulated state.

Network 4: The interoceptive system (the eighth sense)

Sensing the body's internal state via interoceptors inside and around our organs is the essential, life-ensuring task of this system, which tracks everything from our breathing rate and how hungry we are to how full our bladder is. It also detects whether tissue damage has occurred or is likely to occur. This particular type of input is called *nociception*, from the Latin *nocere*, which means 'to harm or to hurt'.

When we notice our heart rate has increased while walking up a hill, that's our interoception system at work. More commonly, though, interoception is more of an inner knowing or sense – think butterflies in the stomach or a 'gut instinct' – than a concrete signal. That said, our interoceptive abilities vary widely. One person might be so hyper aware of their inner system that they can even feel food travelling through their digestive tract (this is a rare example of hypersensitive interoception) while another might not even feel pain while walking on a sprained ankle.

When this system detects an imbalance or need from an organ, it sends messages to the brain, which then replies with orders tailored to address the issue. Too hot? You'll start sweating and your blood vessels will dilate, cooling you down. Thirsty? You'll have an urge to get a drink. Freezing cold? You'll start shivering, which will increase your body temperature, bringing you closer towards your set point.

Together, interoception and exteroception tell the brain whether we're in danger. Though it's common to view the brain as some sort of supercomputer in charge of our emotions, it's actually the 'body-up' signals coming from our three internal networks – proprioception, the vestibular system and interoception – that have the greatest influence over our brain–body system. While we can evaluate the outer world with conscious thought, it's the inner signals that provide the bulk of information the brain uses to determine if we're safe or in danger, and keep our systems and organs functioning as they should. In fact, 80 per cent of the messages whizzing around the vagus nerve, which is a major part of the *interoceptive network*, are being sent *from* the body *to* the brain.

Interoception and body systems

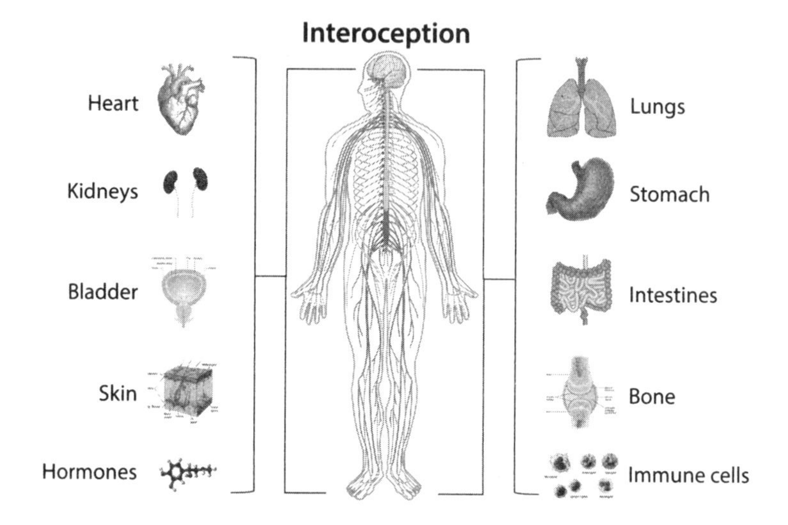

Neuroception

In our analogy of the news corporation, the interoceptive system is the network that needs fact checking – not because its sources or messengers are trying to mislead anyone, but because the messages coming from it aren't as clear as those from the other three networks. Your fingertips, for example, might be able to tell your brain whether something is definitely hot or cold, but your gut can't be nearly as specific.

Consequently, when the brain receives messages from the interoceptive system, it often has to fill in some blanks. It adds information gathered from our exteroceptive system and then makes predictions about how safe or unsafe we are based on what it already knows. If it deems that the people, place or situation in front of us is safe, then we remain in – or move towards – a state where we can connect and enjoy ourselves. If it decides we're in danger, internal alarms go off and we switch immediately into a survival state designed to protect us.

This 'predicting' is known as *neuroception*, which occurs so immediately and outside of our conscious awareness that we're not even aware it's happening, or that we've shifted states.

interoception + exteroception = neuroception

Neuroception determines the nervous system state we shift into and how we respond in any given moment. Neuroception depends a lot on our past experiences, and when our brain misinterprets information or makes the wrong prediction (as it frequently does), we call this faulty neuroception.

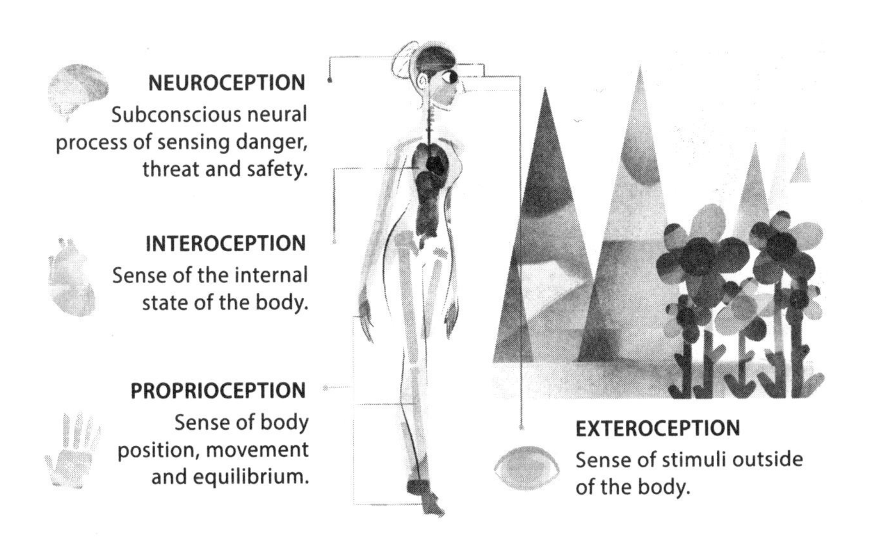

Faulty neuroception

The fact that the human brain is a prediction machine is pretty helpful most of the time. Imagine if you had to be taught how to use a knife and fork every time you sat down for a meal, or had to relearn how to tie your shoes every morning. Instead, you slip on a trainer and bend over, and your brain reads those bodily cues and thinks, *Ooh! I know what comes next. We tie these laces*. Then, without giving the task a second thought, your laces are tied and you're out the door.

The problem with any prediction machine, though, is that sometimes it gets things wrong. Let's say we experience something that's highly activating for us – being bitten by a dog, for example. If we can't discharge the resulting stress in a healthy way (such as those we'll explore in Chapter 9), our brain will learn that dogs = trauma, and it will file away this conclusion for future, along with all of the feelings and nervous system responses we experienced during that attack.

Past experiences make us more sensitive to a similar situation, and traumatic stress conditions us towards more fear and anxiety. So from the day we were bitten, whenever we encounter a dog – even a really gentle one – our brain won't be able to help jumping to the conclusion that this animal is a threat to our safety. As this happens more and more, we'll become conditioned to respond to dogs in this way. This is an example of faulty neuroception, too much of which creates problems.

If we feel a strong fear response or even terror every time we encounter a dog, we'll be in a highly activated state way more often than necessary. Over time, this faulty neuroception may shrink our window of tolerance, making it *even more* likely that we'll experience ongoing or chronic stress outside our window. Adding to this cycle is the fact that we're programmed with an innate negativity bias, which essentially means we tend to think the worst, not the best. This can make it even harder for us to change these patterns – but believe me, they can be changed. That's exactly what we're going to be working on with this nervous system reset.

Scenario 1: Faulty neuroception at work

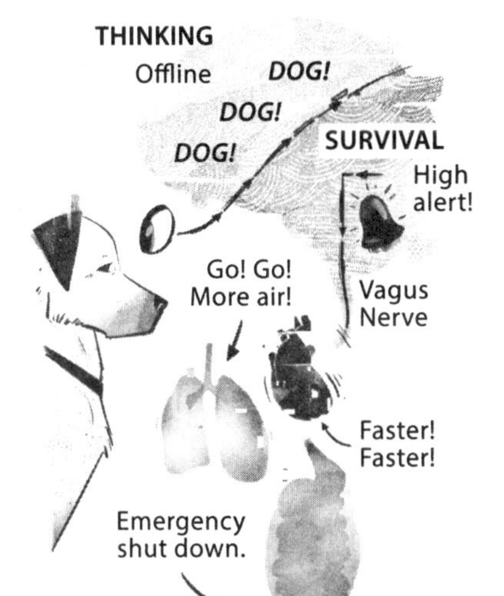

Scenario 2: Regulated neuroception at work

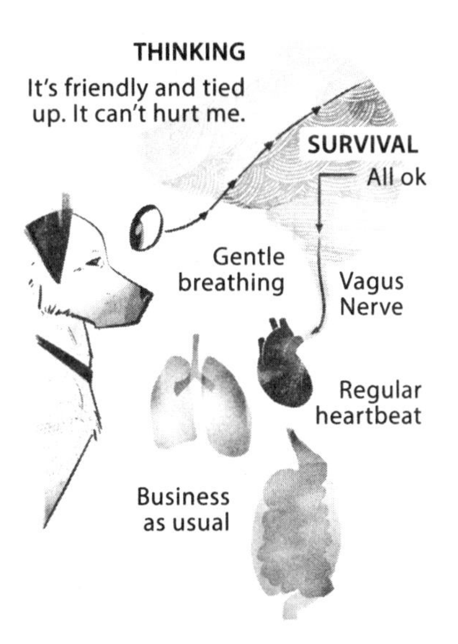

For Sophia, who we met in Chapter 1, the chronic stresses of caring for her terminally ill mother-in-law shrank her window of tolerance to the point that the mere sight of a hospital, something that wouldn't have bothered her in the past, caused her brain to assume that she (or someone she loved) was in danger. The repeated inaccurate signals to her brain reduced her vagal tone still further, increasing her distress.

Thankfully, we can unlearn these patterns not only by training our brain to be better at responding accurately to the stimuli in front of us rather than defaulting to predictions about what's going to happen, but also by training our body to improve the accuracy of its interoception. In Sophia's case, she could retrain her brain–body system to interpret the sight of a hospital as an ordinary, everyday experience by helping herself return to regulation. One way for her to start doing this might be learning to recognise the particular feelings that come up for her when she sees a hospital – a racing heart, for example, and shallow breathing.

When she feels this activation starting, rather than getting overwhelmed and swept away by internal sensations, she might spend a minute consciously focusing on her exteroceptive senses. Noticing the smell of the air, the warmth of the sun on her skin and the mingled sound of birdsong and traffic will give her brain accurate information about what's really happening in her world.

By leaning in to her external world, and reading the cues reality is giving her, she'll be better able to bring herself back to the moment she's in and feel safe. The interrelationship between exteroception and interoception underlies our sense of self and the nervous system state we shift into. This is how we can retrain our nervous system to move from *prediction* to the present moment, and this changes very important memory systems. We'll learn how to do this ourselves in Part Two. Every time we do, our brain–body system learns something new.

By doing this over and over again, Sophia will be beating a new path in the overgrown forest between her body and brain. The first few times will likely be hard going, but every time she walks this new path, it will get easier and clearer, until one day she'll realise that feeling calm when walking near a hospital has become her *new* normal.

Training our brain–body system in this way, and getting better at identifying faulty neuroception and returning to regulation when it occurs, strengthens our vagal tone and expands our window of tolerance. Widening the window makes it much easier for us to face difficult experiences. This is why the training you'll undertake in Part Two is so vital to managing and regulating your nervous system.

Window of tolerance: Narrow vs wide

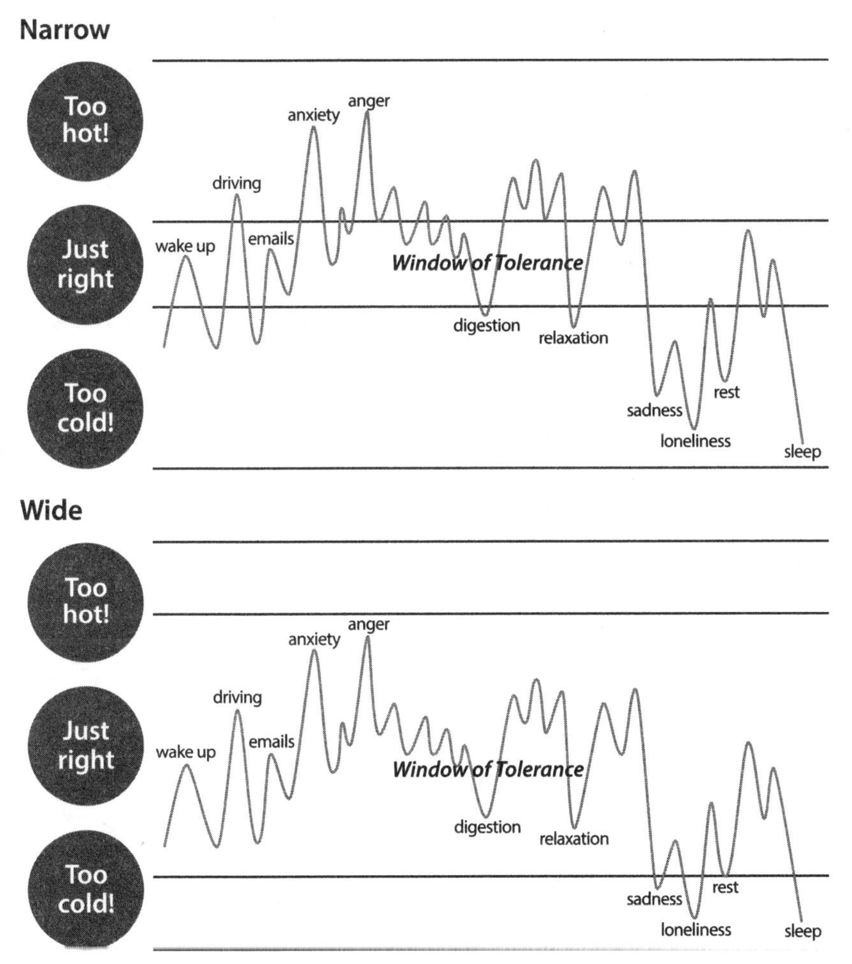

If you frequently find yourself overreacting, or doing things impulsively when you feel anxious, it might be because your window of tolerance has for some reason become narrower. You'll likely benefit a lot from examining how faulty neuroception might be influencing your behaviour. The more you practise building interoceptive awareness and reflecting on how you feel and behave, the easier it becomes to recognise when you're responding to an old trigger rather than your current reality.

Similarly, if you have a tendency to feel empty or numb inside, learning that these feelings are related to dysregulation can go a long way to helping you cope with them. Rather than seeing these feelings as a defect, you can step back and start to challenge your subconscious narratives that you're not enough or unworthy.

Thankfully, we can strengthen our interoceptive skills through training and get better at noticing and interpreting these types of signals when we receive them, resulting in fewer instances of faulty neuroception.

Interoception: 'Too much of anything is a bad thing.'

This saying is true of interoception because while developing good interoception is crucial to being able to regulate our nervous system, too much interoception can be . . . well, too much. There's a reason why so many bodily functions happen automatically, without us being aware of them. It would be so overwhelming if we were aware of *all* the sensory information occurring in our bodies *all* the time. We'd be unable to focus and we'd find it much harder to register those essential signals such as hunger or pain.

Ideally, we want to be skilled enough that we can tune in to our inner world, but not to the point that we register everything all of the time.

Wellbeing and our three internal sense networks

Training the interoceptive system is a priority when resetting the nervous system, because the interoceptive system not only maintains our ideal set point, it also plays a major role in our emotional and mental wellness. An emotion is made up of two or more bodily signals, so it's safe to say that our inner landscape gives rise to our feelings, thoughts and behaviours, and to what's known as our *embodied sense of self.*

Our proprioceptive and vestibular systems play equally important roles in forming this embodied sense of self. They don't just influence our balance in the literal sense, they affect it in an emotional sense, too. When we're regulated, we're likely to feel a sense of agency and control over our life because we have confidence that our body will do the things we want it to. During times of chronic or traumatic stress, however, the messages that these systems send to the brain change, causing us to feel unbalanced physically *and* emotionally. After all, it's hard to feel healthy or in control of your life if you don't have a good sense of where your physical body is in space and you don't feel stable on the ground.

These destabilising feelings can tip us into a state of fight or flight, or make us feel dissociated so that we shut down completely.

How we feel within ourselves based on what our senses are telling us is inextricably linked to who we are and *how* we exist, because the meaning the brain gives our bodily sensations can create emotional distress as well as physical pain.

Eight senses

These eight sensory systems will form the basis of your nervous system reset.

Targeting them can improve your vagal tone, emotional regulation, health and wellbeing, and change how your brain areas communicate when you're stressed. In the chapters to come, you'll soon discover fascinating neuroscience and actionable steps to use in your everyday life.

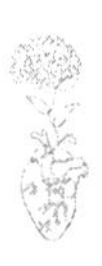

Regardless of how regulated or dysregulated we've been in the past, we can strengthen our interoception skills, retrain our systems to better manage stress, and become emotionally regulated through the process of bioplasticity. First though, we need a roadmap so we can work out where we are, and where we're going.

3

The human nervous system

It's time to zoom out a little now and look at the big picture. Our nervous system is a large, delicately balanced ecosystem comprising several subsystems. It's a bit like an orchestra. Each section is independent but influences all of the others. They must work together to create one harmonious sound – in this case, our wellbeing and survival. How well or poorly each section performs determines the mood, rhythm and tempo of your life, and how well you perform overall.

The more you understand the many ways that chronic stress and trauma can change your physiology, the more likely you'll be to discover that the problem isn't *you*, it's how your nervous system is responding to the world. Like all mammals, our nervous system is an inner surveillance system designed to detect danger via neuroception. If your surveillance system mobilises your energy, creating anxiety that then keeps you awake by playing negative thoughts on a loop, you'll *feel* fearful or upset, no matter what you tell yourself consciously. If you get so burned out by the pressures of life that the weekly grocery shop becomes an impossible task, calling yourself lazy or embarrassing isn't going to fix that or give you the energy to get it done.

You're not too sensitive, needy, anxious, depressed, reactive or co-dependent – your inner system is just trying to keep you safe.

The patterns you've fallen into are adaptive responses of a nervous system that's become oversensitive to cues of danger due to past chronic or traumatic stress. Accepting these patterns as a product of your animal nature and lived experience can do wonders for dissolving deep feelings of shame and blame. As neuroscientist and psychologist Lisa Feldman Barrett says, 'An emotion is your brain's creation of what your bodily sensations mean, in relation to what is going on around you in the world'.

The four fact-finding networks we learned about in the previous chapter – exteroception, proprioception, the vestibular system and interoception – send and receive messages via the two parts of the nervous system – the central nervous system (the brain and spinal cord) and the peripheral nervous system (the body). And as you'll soon see, the two-way communication system that exists between these two systems is absolutely central to how we feel, how healthy we are and how we behave. In this chapter we'll concentrate on the central nervous system; in the next we'll move on to the all-important peripheral nervous system.

The central nervous system

An easy way to remember this system is to think of it as two *central* structures: one in the *centre* of our head (brain), the other running down the *centre* of our body (spinal cord). Within this system, electrical impulses and chemical signals passing from neuron (brain cell) to neuron send information between different areas of the brain and, via the neurons (nerve cells) in nerves, carry information between the brain and the body.

If we picture the entire brain–body system as a world map that you might see at the back of an airline's in-flight magazine, and each key region of the brain as an airport, then the brainstem – the most primitive part of our brain, sitting just above the spine – is a vital airport for connecting flights (the messages) that travel between our body and brain via both our spinal cord and vagus nerve. The planes flying in and out of this airport are the neurons. Those messages travelling upward from the body might hop onto their 'connecting flight' at the brainstem in order to get to different airports throughout the brain. This impacts our emotions, learning, cognition and thoughts in the process.

There are billions of neurons in our body, and they vary in structure, function and genetic makeup. For example, sensory neurons help us taste, smell, hear, see and feel, while motor neurons help us move – voluntarily and involuntarily. Neurons allow the brain and spinal cord to communicate with muscles, organs and glands all over the body.

Interestingly, the brain itself is not made up of just neurons. There are blood vessels, of course, and in some regions of the brain there are more immune cells than there are neurons. Neurons and

THE NERVOUS SYSTEM

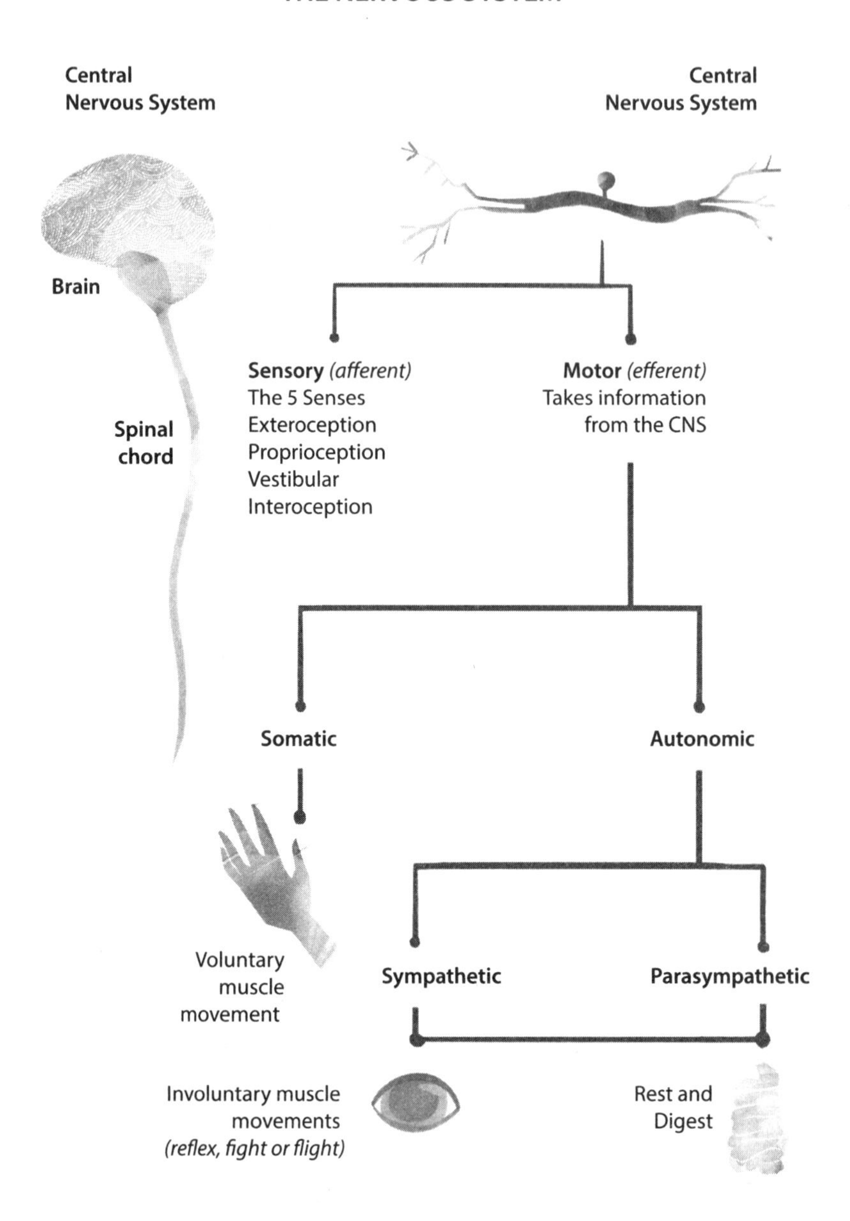

immune cells are so closely interconnected that they rely on each other to work. Together, they make up the neuroimmune system.

The brain

The brain has long been viewed as the commander of the body, but that doesn't accurately describe its role. Many important instructions are, of course, sent from the brain to the body – brain-down signals, if you will – but the body-up signals sent by our internal sensory and neural networks actually help the brain decide what those orders should be. Our brains didn't evolve for logical thinking, happiness or accuracy. All brains are here for the same mission: to make sure there are enough resources for our body's systems so that we can survive and reproduce. We learned about this earlier when you were introduced to allostasis (see page 8).

When we start tuning in to our nervous system using interoception, and track it by noticing the physical sensations and movements of our body, we're engaging those all-important body-up signals. By learning to use both of these pathways – body-up and brain-down, we'll be building regulation and stabilising the body's sensations and impulses.

From conception, our brain develops in a fairly linear way. Think of this development as like a staircase, where each step represents a phase of physical brain development. Early in the womb, the brainstem develops to form the bottom step, then more steps are added before birth and then rapidly throughout childhood. It's believed that 90 per cent of brain development happens before the age of five. Around age 25, the top stair forms and we reach the apex of this staircase, which is a fully formed prefrontal cortex.

To simplify this incredibly complex organ, we often divide the brain into two main parts: the *thinking brain* (the cortex) and the *survival brain* (the brainstem, cerebellum and limbic system). Their names sum up their primary functions, but it's important to note that they don't exist as two solitary islands within our head. There's a constant flow of two-way communication between them, just as there is between our body and brain. So although we'll be referring to them this way throughout the book, it's worth noting that our experience of bodily sensations, pain and emotions involves large networks that expand across *both* of these areas.

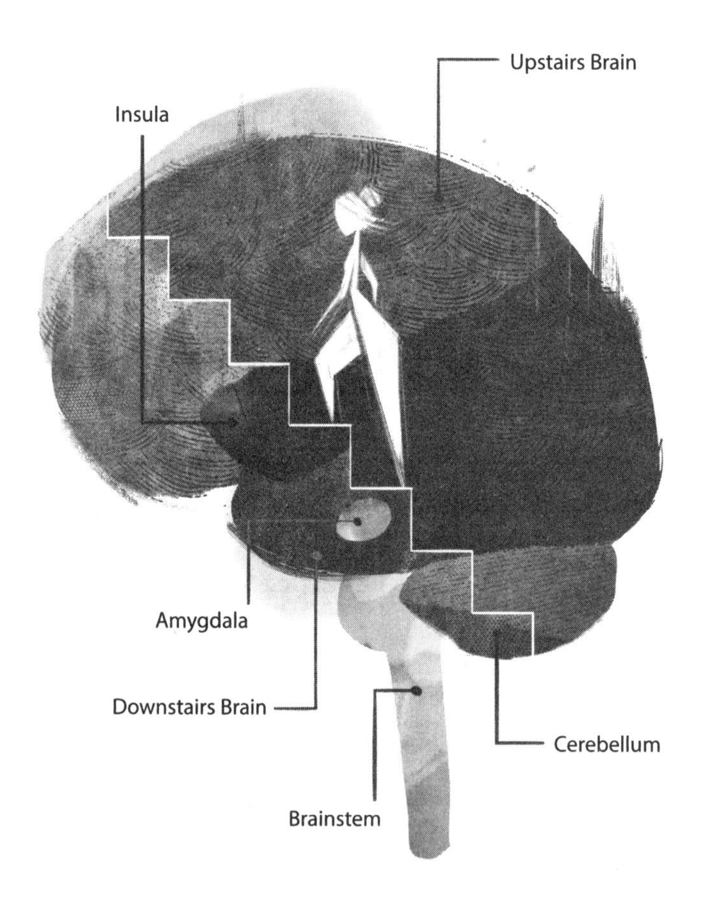

Survival brain (aka lower brain)

This includes the brainstem, cerebellum (Latin for 'little brain') and limbic system. These are the first parts of the brain to develop, and they play an important role in regulating the systems that keep us alive, such as our breathing and heartbeat.

Information from the sensory systems help this brain detect whether a situation is safe or dangerous. As it processes the various messages it's gathering, it *predicts* what's going to happen and quickly triggers an appropriate nervous system response. These predictions are based on the survival brain's memory system, which stores 'implicit' memories (memories we're not aware of and can't access consciously, also called unconscious or automatic memory) that help us make sense of the world and learn skills to navigate it in the future. It may not remember who you were with or the day you learned to ride a bike, but the bodily memories it stored during that experience are the reason you can hop on a bike today without having to relearn how to balance yourself as you pedal. After my daughter was born, I was amazed by the number of nursery rhymes I could remember from my own childhood!

Implicit learning involves neuroception (which to recap is exteroception plus interoception) – which happens when bodily signals (interoception) and our five senses (exteroception) send information to the survival brain. Within the limbic system, the amygdala is our internal fire alarm, while the cerebellum and basal ganglia are our implicit memory database, storing information in case we encounter something similar again. In most cases, the predictions from our survival brain are sent upstairs to our thinking brain (on those connecting flights I mentioned earlier). Ideally, the thinking brain considers the prediction and gathers additional information to determine whether that prediction is valid or incorrect. But when we're under stress, the brain prioritises efficiency and safety, so we may lose sight of the big picture, shift outside our window of tolerance and simply react.

How stress impacts the survival brain

When we're dysregulated and experiencing strong emotions, there's more activity (blood flow) in our survival brain regions. The higher regions of the brain (the thinking brain) may also go offline, closing their airports to those connecting flights from the lower brain. Following trauma, specific motor areas in the survival brain are often activated, which explains why our body tightens or shifts instinctively without us realising it. When we connect back with our body after a stressful time, we may notice just how much we've been clenching our jaw or bracing through our rib cage. Our posture can give us many clues about which state we're in and, as you'll see in the coming chapters, it can also be a doorway back to regulation.

Thinking brain (aka higher brain)

Also known as the cerebrum, the thinking brain includes important regions such as the prefrontal cortex, which exerts a downregulating or calming influence on the survival brain by suppressing the stress response and playing a role in the regulation of the stress hormone cortisol.

Our thinking brain helps us think rationally, plan for the future and use language, logic and creativity. Like the survival brain, it stores memories, but these memories are far more detailed – we call them explicit memories because we can recall them consciously. These are the stories that you tell or the holidays you think of fondly. In the example of learning to ride a bike, your thinking brain can remember who taught you, and what the weather was like when you finally mastered this skill.

The areas of the brain involved with explicit memories are the hippocampus and the amygdala, and these memories are later stored in higher brain regions when we sleep.

The thinking brain is also responsible for conscious movement. When we get up from a chair or pick something up, it's because a region in our thinking brain called the motor cortex has been activated. This is a little different from the way our body reflexively braces or collapses when we move out of our window of tolerance, or when we go into a closed posture in response to conflict.

Implicit and explicit memories

Traumatic events are often stored in the body as implicit memories. These are fragments of memory that return with strong feelings (e.g. intense fear), sensations (e.g. restriction in the chest) and movements (e.g. clenching our jaw and fists), which have been stored since the time of the original trauma and are now being experienced again in the present. We're usually unable to put these experiences into words and this is why we want to use our sensory systems to transform them into explicit memories – they become part of our story, not something we relive.

How stress impacts the thinking brain

Under high levels of stress, activity in our thinking brain tends to slow and our rational brain may temporarily go offline. When that happens, sensory information from the body gets interrupted on its way to the thinking brain – the plane is grounded partway through its journey. Consequently, we may feel destabilised, overwhelmed, disconnected or even unable to pinpoint or define what we're feeling. In these instances, reconnecting with our body – as we'll learn to do in Part Two – is critical to actively managing these emotions and restoring a sense of balance. We do this by integrating brain-down and body-up information, which will return us to regulation, flow and ease.

As we saw earlier, mindset strategies alone can't change our physiology or emotional reactions if we're dysregulated. But if we're not aware of this and we keep trying to change our nervous system state by using thinking-brain strategies like minimising what we feel in our body and telling ourselves, *It's not that bad*, or comparing ourselves to others, *Kate's got it so much worse than me*, we might feel like a failure when we're still feeling anxious, agitated, angry or shutdown. And then our inner critic might get louder – leading to even more activation. Telling yourself to *Suck it up*, *Just get on with it*, or *Soldier on* won't change the nervous system's autonomic threat-detection system, because that exists in our survival brain *not* our thinking brain. For change to happen, we need to work with the body's sensory systems through bottom-up interventions, as they're the ones speaking the language of the survival brain.

The primary language centre, known as Broca's area, is also located in the thinking brain, just near our left ear. It's thought to be responsible for translating our personal experiences into communicable language. Several studies have shown that under high levels of stress Broca's area goes offline, and this explains why talking about our distress is not the best practice. Encouraging people to talk about what's happened to them when they're dysregulated can increase their frustration, leading to more stress arousal and disconnection from the body.

Since the survival brain informs the thinking brain, one way we can work with these 'lower steps' is through body-up regulation. For one thing, focusing on the body can provide us with a feeling of safety and stability. Awareness of our muscles and joints, the grounded sensation of our feet on the floor, or the centring we feel as we tune in to our belly, can bring a whole new dimension to our embodied sense of self that tells us who we are and how we're doing. It's also more productive, when we're already overwhelmed and struggling to understand our emotions, than focusing on worrying thoughts. For many of us, giving these worries more airtime only increases our ruminating (dwelling) on these thoughts and our anxiety.

The spinal cord

The second part of the central nervous system is the spinal cord, which begins at the bottom of the brainstem and ends at the tailbone in the lower back. The spinal nerves spreading out from this cord form part of our peripheral nervous system (so called because it communicates with the parts of the body on the periphery, i.e. outside, the central nervous system; see Chapter 4). The spinal nerves carry sensations, for example, from the skin to the spinal cord, which then transmits them up to the brain. Receptors in the body also send information – such as that proprioceptive information about where our body parts are at any given moment – up the spinal cord to the brainstem and survival brain.

The spinal cord is crucial to voluntary movement (i.e. conscious movement we can control), which we know can be a powerful source of regulation. It also plays an important role in pain signals. Because of this, it can become hypersensitive to pain cues if past experiences or trauma have 'trained' us to expect pain.

The insula

Deep within our brain sits one of the busiest, most essential airports: the insula. This central airport integrates information from the thinking brain, the survival brain *and* the brainstem. How we perceive our body, our feelings and the outside world depends, therefore, on how the insula and other regions of our thinking brain process the information they receive.

The insula, also known as the insular cortex, plays an incredibly important role in regulating our bodily systems and therefore our nervous system. By practising interoception – by using tools to tune in to your nervous system state – you'll be engaging the insula, which will help you stay connected to your sense of self. Because this central airport connects to our survival brain as well as our thinking brain, when the pathways between the insula and the thinking brain are open and information flows freely between them, our frontal lobe can appraise sensory information more objectively and uncouple it from the fearful or anxious thought with which our survival brain may have learned to link it.

When we fly into that 'hot' survival state, however, those pathways shut down and prevent us from thinking logically. This is why interoceptive training is so important: it keeps key regions of the brain online so we can still see the big picture. When we can recognise what's going on inside us and identify what we need to calm ourselves, we can reopen those pathways and bring our thinking brain back online.

Re-regulation is happening now

One thing I want to stress early on is that your nervous system reset is already underway. There are exercises and tools coming up, of course, but every time you've caught yourself wondering, *What am I feeling? Can I* notice *any messages coming from my body?* you've been strengthening your interoceptive abilities. Since reading about the three different states in Chapter 1, you've probably had at least a handful of moments where you've thought, *What state am I in?* And just that fleeting, simple act of taking your emotional temperature is an indication that you're strengthening your vagal tone and taking a more comprehensive approach to your wellbeing.

Interoception, the insula and extraordinary performance

In 2012, researchers released findings of a study that compared the brains of a group of elite adventure racers with those of a group of healthy subjects. Faced with the same physical stressors, adventure racers were able to perform tasks better than the control group. Brain scans showed more activity (blood flow) in the insulas of the athletes than of the volunteers. This indicated that the athletes had more efficient interoceptive functioning than the control group. They were better able to tune in to the signals from their body and send the insula more accurate information about the situation they were in, thereby minimising the chances that their brain would mistake the stressor for real danger and trigger responses that would cause their performance to falter.

Similar observations were made during a study of elite US Navy SEALs that compared their response to stimuli with that of healthy non-military men their age. Each man was shown positive or negative images. While anticipating a negative image, SEALs were better able to activate the emotional control centre (middle insula) of their brain than the other men. The authors of the study on adventure racers concluded that the insular cortex 'appears to be emerging as an important brain system for optimal performance in extreme environments'.

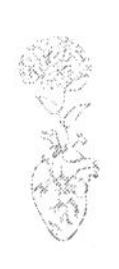

As we saw earlier in this chapter, the central nervous system communicates with the body via the peripheral nervous system. Now let's take a deeper look at the peripheral nervous system and in particular the vagus nerve – the key to the nervous system reset.

4

The peripheral nervous system and the vagus nerve

As the word 'periphery' suggests, this branch of the nervous system is more expansive than the central nervous system, because it includes the billions of nerves that spread out from the spinal cord to every extremity of the body, as well as the vagus nerve. The eight senses from the four sensory systems we met in Chapter 2 feed information to the brain on a continual basis via the peripheral nervous system, which helps us perceive our external environment and understand our reality. This system also keeps the brain updated on our various internal systems, even though we're not aware of the exchange of much of this information.

The peripheral system is made up of two branches – the sensory system (via what are called afferent nerves) and the motor system (via efferent nerves). Each of these has its own subsystems.

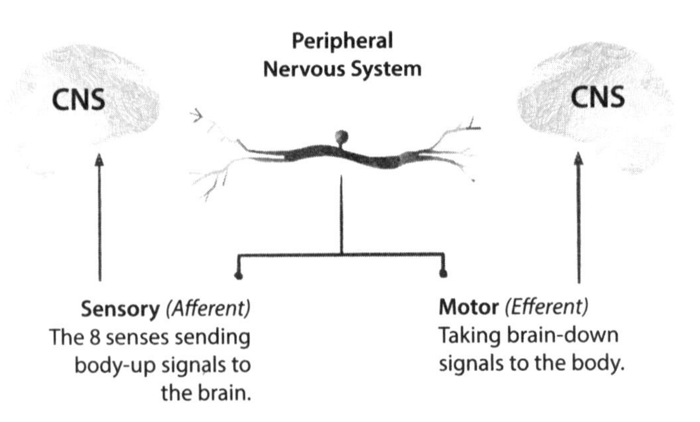

The sensory system

This remarkable part of the peripheral nervous system transmits information gathered from the four fact-finding networks. These exteroceptive, proprioceptive, vestibular and interoceptive systems feed information from the body *towards* the brain (aka body-up) via afferent nerves, which are named for the Latin verb *affere*, meaning 'to bring to'.

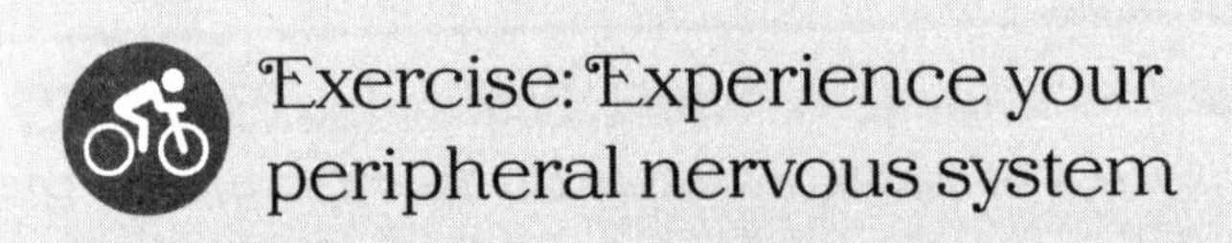

Exercise: Experience your peripheral nervous system

What better way to learn about this branch of your peripheral nervous system than to experience it in action? Let's start by bringing your attention to your hands, then expand to other parts of the body as you consider these questions:

- What does this book or tablet feel like? Is it warm or cool? Heavy or light?

- What can you sense on your skin – the material of your clothing or the pressure of the chair against your back?
- What's the temperature like in this room?
- Is there a breeze?
- What can you smell?
- What sounds can you hear?
- Without looking, can you notice where your feet are in relation to your body?
- How are you holding your head?
- Are your shoulders and neck tense or relaxed?
- Are you sitting up straight or are you slumped over?
- How is your breathing?
- Are you hungry, thirsty, tired or restless? Do you need to go to the bathroom, perhaps?

As you just experienced, a huge amount of exteroceptive and interoceptive information is being relayed to your brain at any given moment, even when you're not aware of it. All of this (and much more that you didn't tune in to) helps your brain predict the immediate future – that neuroception (exteroception + interoception) we talked about in Chapter 2. You may want to make a note of your answers in your notebook or journal, to refer to later.

Remember, a lot of the time our brain makes accurate predictions. But sometimes it doesn't, and when it gets things wrong it's usually because traumatic events or chronic stress have 'taught' our neuroceptive system to become *more* protective and sensitised to danger cues.

The motor system

In contrast to the sensory division, this system carries information *from* the brain *down* to the body (aka brain-down) via efferent nerves – from the Latin *effere*, meaning 'to bring *away* from'. This division of the peripheral nervous system is divided into two further subsystems: the *somatic* nervous system and the *autonomic* nervous system.

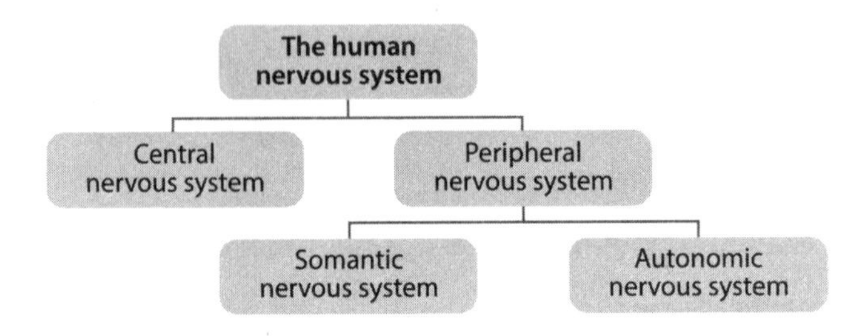

The somatic nervous system

The Latin word for 'body' is *soma*, which is useful to remember, since this is the nervous system we're engaging whenever our body takes conscious physical action. If you want to kick a ball, grab a glass or jump into a lake, your brain and spinal cord send the instructions to the relevant muscles to help them move.

Our body stores our experiences – good and bad – in our survival brain, and encodes it as muscle memory via our proprioceptive senses. This is why, when we experience danger, our muscles contract in ways that change our posture, movements and actions, often without us realising it's happening. For example, clenching your fists and hunching your shoulders can shift you into a hot or cold state, while relaxing your shoulders and smiling can help you feel safe and even return you to regulation. The training (which I prefer to call bioplasticity tools) I'll be sharing with you in Part Two will teach you how to use this subconscious connection – consciously.

The autonomic nervous system

In Latin, *autonomic* means 'involuntary' or 'unconscious', which is exactly how this nervous system operates – on autopilot – sending messages from the survival brain to the body to focus on either survival or recovery.

Once you understand how this system works and build what's known as *autonomic awareness*, you'll be in a much better position to not only cope with stressors in the moment, but also recover from them way quicker and get back to your set point. As you make your way through this book, I hope you'll get better at identifying the patterns you've fallen into, and the many ways your nervous system has been shaped by your past. You'll also become more mindful that what you experience *today* (deliberately or not) is shaping your future stress responses, relationships and more.

The autonomic system is typically divided into two branches: the *sympathetic* nervous system and the *parasympathetic* nervous system.

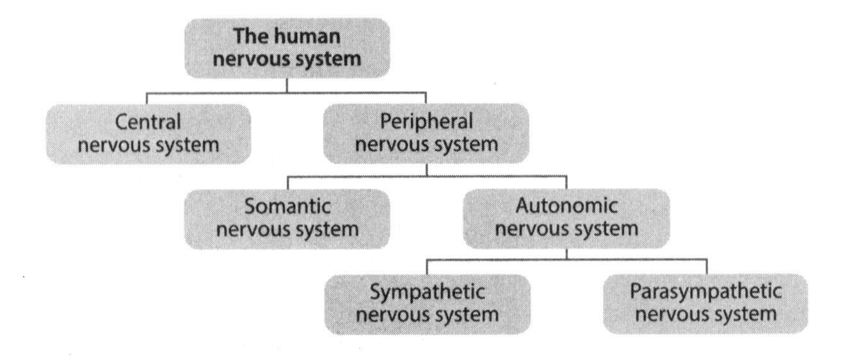

The sympathetic nervous system

This is the system that triggers the shift into the too hot state (also known as the *sympathetic state*). It turns on our survival fight-or-flight responses and mobilises precious energy so we can respond to dangerous situations quickly and effectively. Like a guard dog programmed to keep us safe, this system is constantly scanning for danger, and it responds to perceived threats so instinctively we might not even know a reaction is coming.

We're going to be focusing on this inner surveillance system a lot, because it learns from our past and present experiences, and tries to protect us better in the future. And though that's a very good thing, in some cases it can become *overly* sensitive – like an overprotective guard dog that barks at everyone – and when this happens, it can do more harm than good.

The parasympathetic nervous system

You might have heard this branch of the system referred to as rest and digest. This is the system that keeps everything running smoothly, from our heartbeat and blood flow, to our breathing and digestion. Since all of these processes happen outside of our conscious awareness, this system is sometimes called the involuntary nervous system.

The parasympathetic nervous system also calms our body and conserves energy after a stressful event by slowing our heart, optimising digestion, and lowering blood pressure.

Bodily responses in the sympathetic and parasympathetic state

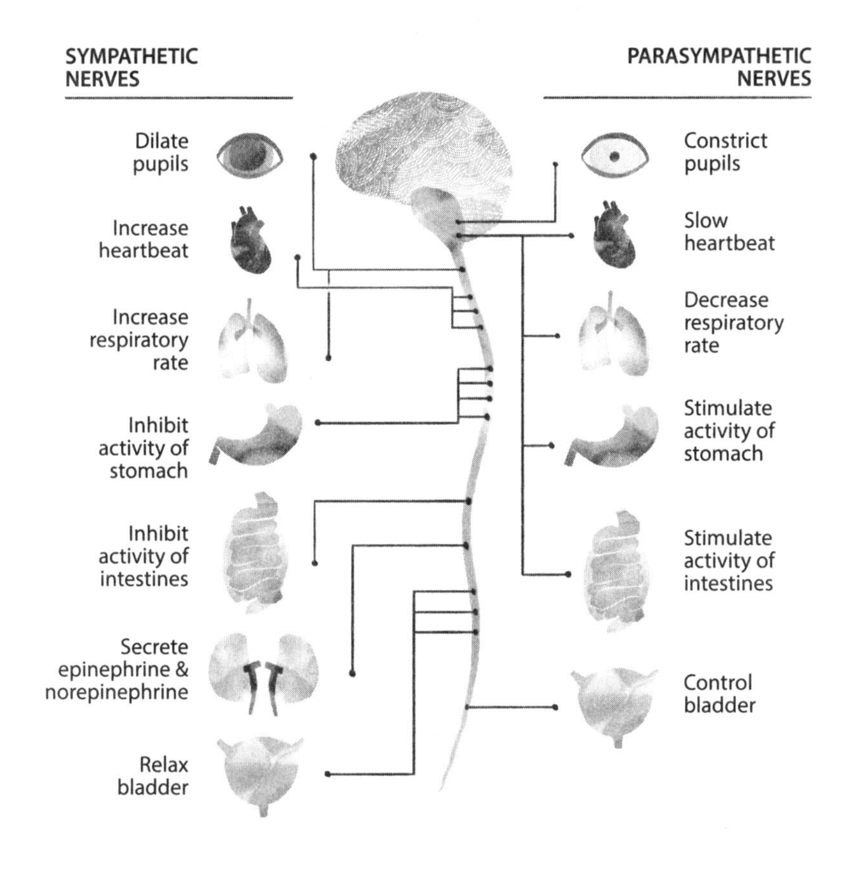

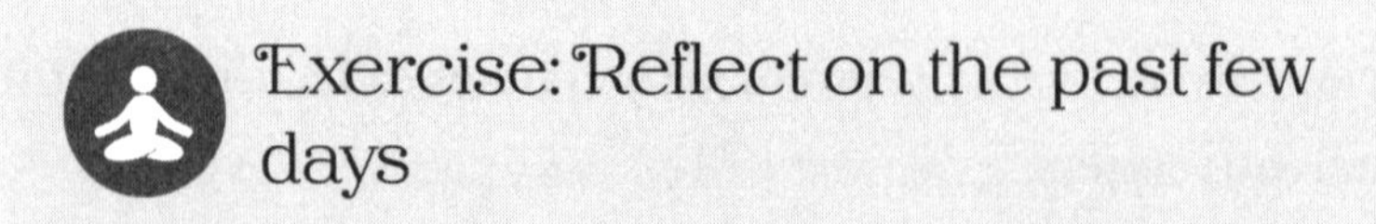

Exercise: Reflect on the past few days

Let's take a moment to think about interoception right now. Look at the image on page 101 and think back about the last couple of days, or even week. Have you noticed yourself experiencing any of the sensations listed? If so, can you recall what was going on for you in those moments? Being able to recognise these changes, either in the moment or after the fact, can give you clues as to which system you're engaging with during those times.

Bearing those responses in mind, the next time you notice a dry mouth, churning stomach, tightness in your chest or a restriction of breath, see if you can pinpoint which nervous system – sympathetic or parasympathetic – is driving those sensations, and try to identify the event or feeling that activated that system. Knowing the events that trigger these types of responses will help you learn to face that particular trigger while staying within your stretch zone (those areas at the edge of your window of tolerance; see page 31), or give yourself space after the event to come back to a regulated state.

If, for example, riding in a crowded commuter train in the morning raises your heartbeat and makes you feel anxious and sweaty, you'll know from the diagram on page 101 that your commute is activating your sympathetic nervous system. Since this happens on a regular basis, it's worth training your body not to perceive this event as threatening by finding ways to make your train journey more pleasant so you can stay within your window of tolerance.

To do that, you might try focusing on early signs of tension as soon as you feel them begin to take hold, either on your way to the train or while you're on it. If you notice that your fists are clenched, actively relax them and wiggle your fingers. If your jaw is tight, try opening and closing your mouth to help it relax. Are you standing rigidly against the door? Does shifting your weight from one foot to the other help? Activating your interoceptive and peripheral nervous systems through this body awareness and voluntary movement engages the vagus nerve and can help you shift back within your window of tolerance.

If it's the crowds of people that bother you, perhaps you can change seats, stand for a while or move to a carriage where you won't feel as stuck or trapped. If not, perhaps you could give yourself permission to get off at the next stop and take a few minutes' break before getting back on again. Any of these things will reassure your nervous system that you have choice or agency in the matter, and the nervous system loves choice.

If these 'in the moment' tactics don't work, consider how you might be able to experience fewer instances of this particular stressor. Could you leave the house 30 minutes earlier to avoid the rush? If not, then look for ways to bring your body back to regulation as quickly as possible after each commute. You could, for example, get off the train one stop early and walk to your destination to give your body and brain time to discharge stress activation and come back to balance.

You may want to make a note in your notebook or journal of what worked and didn't work for you in your particular example, so that next time you encounter the same situation or the same responses, you can try those same tactics again.

The vagus nerve

Appropriately named for the Latin word for 'wandering', the vagus nerve runs from the base of the skull to the depths of the intestines. It comprises many different fibres, 80 per cent of which are afferent (carrying signals to the brain), and the remainder efferent (carrying signals from the brain to the body) (see image on page 22).

This information superhighway is comparable in size to the spinal cord, and although it has a single name, it's really an entire system of its own. At the brainstem, there are two main branches, the ventral vagus nerve and the dorsal vagus nerve. The ventral vagus nerve connects to structures above the diaphragm (the face, neck, chest and lungs), while the dorsal vagus nerve connects to the organs in the abdomen. In the chest, these two branches subdivide into a cosmos of nerves that span our lungs, heart, diaphragm, stomach, spleen, intestines, colon, liver and kidneys. This network of nerves beams millions of messages to and from the brain, maintaining regulation and sending signals of pain, danger or safety.

The vagus nerve is a *major* part of the brain–body connection.

Polyvagal theory

In 1995, Dr Stephen Porges, director at the time of the Brain-Body Center at the University of Illinois in Chicago, posited a theory poised to expand our understanding of the vagus nerve and the role it plays in our health and emotional wellbeing. This polyvagal theory suggested firstly that the two branches of the vagal nerve played very different roles, and secondly that the autonomic nervous system has three states rather than two. These three states – the sympathetic (too hot) and two states within the parasympathetic nervous system called the ventral vagal (just-right) and dorsal vagal (too cold) states – can be used to understand how we react to stress and trauma.

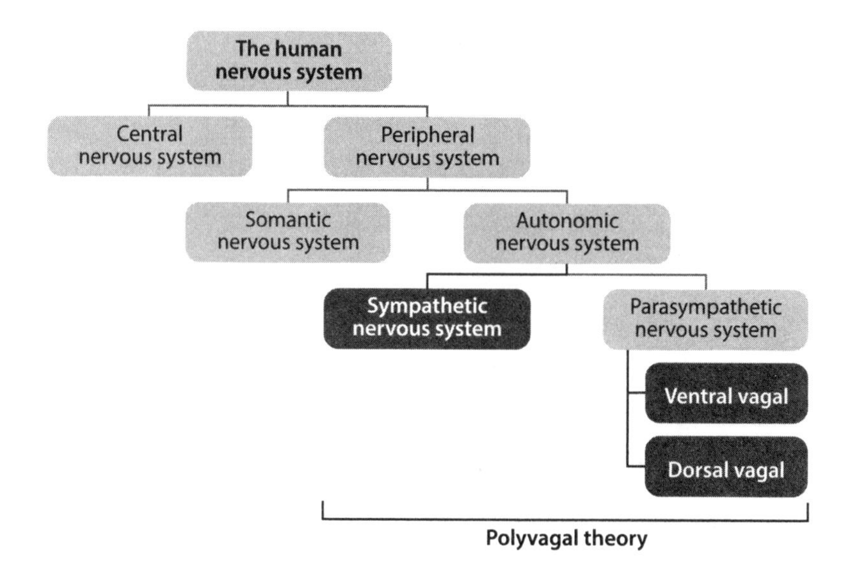

The ventral vagal branch

This more recently evolved branch of the vagus nerve gives rise to our just-right state – known in polyvagal theory as the ventral vagal state – and helps us return to regulation. It originates in the brainstem, travels down through the neck and throat with branches spreading out to the ears, and supplies nerves to the heart and lungs as well as structures and organs above the diaphragm – the oesophagus and the bronchi of the lungs, as well as the larynx and pharynx, which are involved with speech and communication. This branch of the vagus nerve is myelinated. This means that, like many nerves, it's covered in a fatty insulative coating similar to plastic insulation around electrical wires that helps it function quickly and accurately.

The dorsal vagal branch

This division of the vagus nerve plays an important role in maintaining good digestion and contributes to healthy homeostasis. It also acts to slow down our physiology, but because this more primitive branch of the vagus nerve is not myelinated – i.e. there's no insulation around this electrical wiring – the signals it transmits aren't as accurate or as finely tuned as those whizzing around the ventral vagal branch. Consequently, Porges theorised, in the face of a threat, it's likely to take us into the too cold nervous system state – known in polyvagal theory as the dorsal vagal state.

Nerve cells

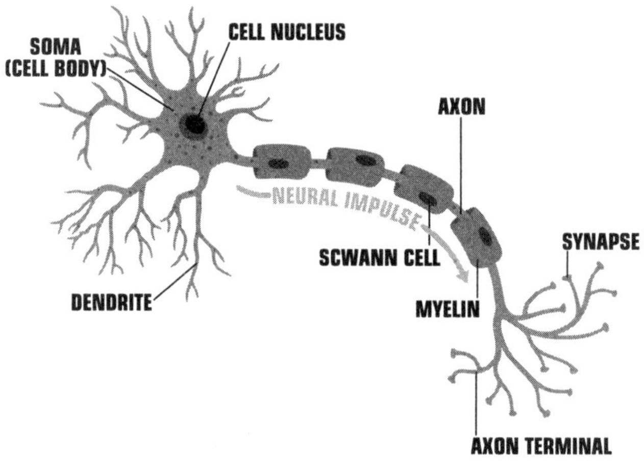

Neurons are the brain cells and nerve cells found throughout the human body. There are numerous types of neurons, but the basic plan is illustrated above. The main body of the nerve cell has branching extensions at the top called dendrites. These form connections with other nerve cells. At the bottom of the cell body is a long extension called an axon, which in many nerve cells is covered by a myelin sheath. At the end of the axon are more branches, which reach out and end in synapses, which pass messages in the form of neurotransmitters to the dendrites of other nerve cells.

The dorsal vagal branch also originates in the brain stem and travels under the diaphragm, but there it branches out like a vine and spreads right down to the colon. The axons (nerve cell tails; see box) of dorsal vagal neurons carry information over long distances. If we're feeling safe and connected, the dorsal vagal branch immobilises our physiology and we move into stillness, but under threat it acts as a handbrake and causes us to freeze or shut down.

Polyvagal theory in action

In summary, polyvagal theory posits three possible nervous system states, which match up with the three nervous system states we already know from Chapter 1:

1. Sympathetic state = too hot state
2. Ventral vagal state = just-right state
3. Dorsal vagal state = too cold state

For simplicity, I'll continue referring to these three states as hot, cold and just right for the most part, but they're one in the same. We now know that the constant loop of messages flowing between the brain and body via the vagus nerve is responsible for keeping our internal thermostat regulated and allows us to respond to situations as they arise.

When the interoceptive messages coming from our organs relate to maintaining homeostasis and are updates on specific vital statistics (such as pH levels, heartbeat or blood pressure), the brain can discern where those messages have come from and what they're about with remarkably high precision, and responds in equally specific ways.

This echoes the way our smartphones can parse a broad range of information. Throughout the day, your phone not only notifies you every time someone communicates with you, it also tells you *who* is trying to reach you, what mode of communication they're using (calling, texting, DMing, etc.) *and* what number, account or email address they're contacting you from. In addition to those notifications, you might also receive dozens of notifications from apps, each with their own specific uses and functions, and likely also with their own unique notification sound. Just like your phone, your brain sorts information from a broad range of inputs as it comes in. But *how* does it do this?

Part of the answer lies in the neurons of the vagus nerve. There are body-up vagus neurons and brain-down vagus neurons, and these carry coded information in their electrical signals. This coding, which still isn't well understood, enables a high level of precision, and tells the brain:

- which organ the signal is coming from
- which tissue layer *within* the organ the signal is arising from
- what the stimulus is.

Researchers believe that there are different groups of neurons in the vagus nerve with similar genetic properties that each detect a particular type of stimulus. Genetic codes for organ information have also been discovered in the vagus nerve. This means that specific messages can be sent from one location, such as the intestines, to inform the brain about, say, the release of hormones, inflammation or mechanical pressure. Even though this cluster of data comes from the same location, the way it's coded means that within the brain it can be refined and separated with granularity. This is how the brain knows exactly who's 'calling' and what they want. The exception to this occurs when we're triggered (usually unconsciously) by stress or trauma. In these cases, the bodily sensations and responses tied to that faulty neuroception create broad, diffuse messages of distress or danger that our brain finds much harder to decipher.

Though most of this interoception happens without our knowledge, we can help our brain–body system function more optimally by learning how to influence certain body-up signals.

For instance, by deliberately changing our breathing pattern to stretch our lungs, we can send signals to the brainstem and change our nervous system state.

The vagus nerve is an intricate and finely tuned bidirectional system, and that two-way communication is the reason the vagus nerve plays such a key role in our emotional and physical health. It is intricately connected to our moods, immune response, digestion, heart rate, breathing rate, cardiovascular functioning, and reflexes such as coughing, sneezing, swallowing and vomiting. It's easy to see why dysregulation of the nervous system, in which the vagus nerve plays a major part, can create ongoing issues in our brain and body.

When we prioritise having a healthy, functioning vagus nerve – with good vagal tone – we are more likely to have a resilient and adaptable nervous system. Research has shown an association between high vagal tone and improved health and improved emotional state and cognition.

You can work on increasing your vagal tone using the resources in Part Two of this book. This will allow you to influence those body-up messages, freeing you from some of your most distressing emotional and physical struggles. Improved vagal tone makes us better at getting ourselves unstuck when we experience anxiety, anger, despair or apathy, and leaves us better equipped to maintain our equilibrium in the future, even in the face of adversity.

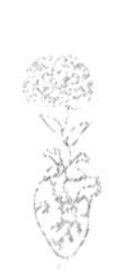

In the next chapter we'll look in more detail at the brain–body and body–brain communication within the vagus nerve, and at how this affects our health and wellbeing.

5

The body-up, brain-down loop

As we've seen, the two-way communication between the brain and body is what makes the vagus nerve one of the most influential structures in our body. Our moods and our thoughts, not to mention our immune response, digestion, heart rate, breathing rate and cardiovascular functioning are all tied to this nerve.

As part of the autonomic system, much of this communication via the vagus nerve goes unnoticed within our body. While we eat, sleep, play and argue, our brain is in constant communication with our internal organs, and those body-up electrical signals whizzing through the vagus nerve from each organ are what help the brain monitor our health and maintain homeostasis. Some organs, however, wield more influence than others, which is why we'll suddenly become aware of a racing heart or butterflies in our tummy if we move into a hotter state. In this chapter, we'll explore the profound effect that the heart, gut and fascia (the web of connective tissue around our muscles, blood vessels and nerves) have on our mental and emotional state as well as our physical health.

The heart–brain axis

Two of the most important pieces of information the brain receives about the body are heartbeat and blood pressure. As with every other part of the body, communication between the brain and the heart operates as a constant bidirectional feedback loop, but the heart has distinctive features that allow it to be in constant communication with the brain. This particular feedback loop is often referred to as the heart–brain axis.

The vagus nerve sends signals to the brain from baroreceptors (pressure sensors) on the heart walls, the aortic arch (which sits above the heart and links the upward and downward branches of the aorta, the body's main artery) and the carotid bodies (near the carotid arteries in the neck; see diagram below). These three sets of baroreceptors help our body keep our blood pressure at a relatively constant level so that blood continues pumping up to our brain no matter which position we're in.

Baroreceptors

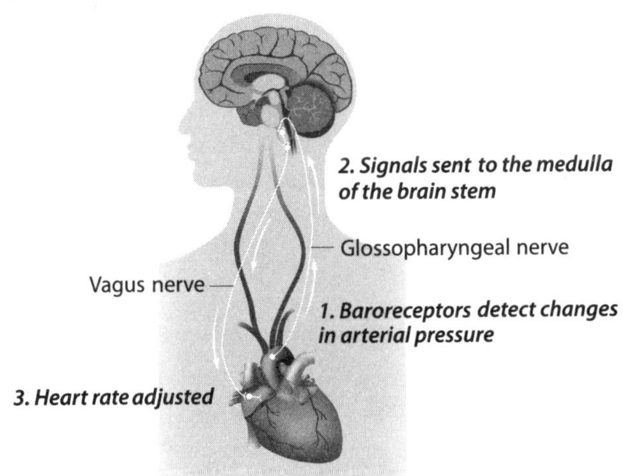

When we get out of bed in the morning and stand up, for example, the necessary increase in blood pressure stretches our baroreceptors, creating a shift in the brain–body system as it tries to maintain homeostasis. These baroreceptors also register the activity of the heart, which in turn influences how we feel and act. If our heart is beating quickly, for example, they send signals that our brain might register as a sense of fight or flight.

The vagal brake

Within the heart is an incredibly important structure called the sinoatrial node. It's tiny but mighty, and is commonly referred to as the heart's pacemaker. The vagus nerve is directly connected to this pacemaker via a pathway known as the *vagal brake*, which is another crucial part of our biology, and one designed to help us survive.

The sinoatrial node and vagus nerve

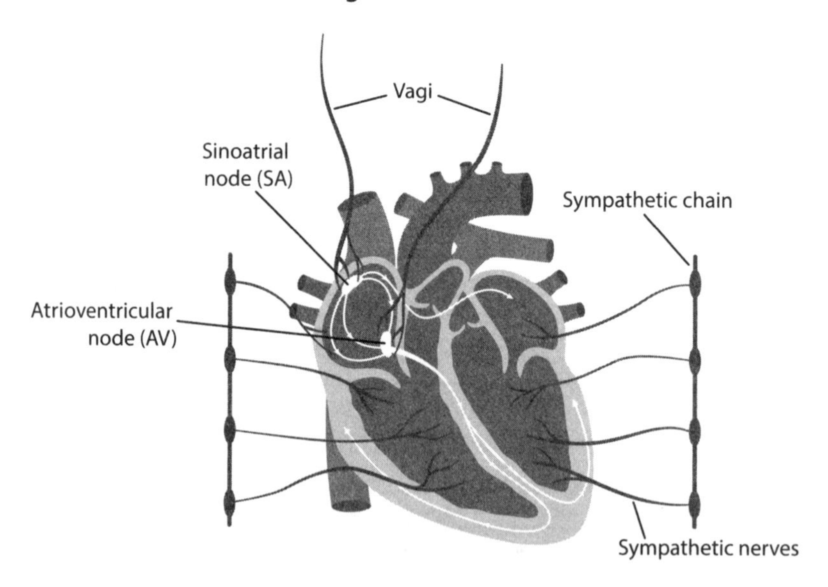

In a similar way to brakes on a bike or car, our vagal brake can be engaged and released to alter the speed of our heartbeat. When we're in the 'too cold' dorsal vagal state, the immobilising energy can slow the heart to as few as 20–30 beats a minute or even stop it completely. Without the vagal brake, the average resting heartbeat would be up between 90 and 110 beats per minute rather than the standard 72 beats per minute.

Nervous System mechanics

We can think of our nervous system as a car. The mobilising sympathetic energy is the accelerator or gas. The ventral branch is the brake pedal we use with our foot. The dorsal vagal branch is like putting on the handbrake and immobilises us.

If you reflect on the things you do on a daily or weekly basis and consider the ways your brake either releases or engages, you'll get a good idea of how much flexibility it gives you, and how useful it can be. On the way to a date, for example, your vagal brake is likely to release a little, making you a touch more energetic, engaging and confident. The same applies during a job interview or other important meeting. By easing up on that brake, your body is giving you access to that hotter energy so you can reap the benefits of a boosted personality and increased focus. If you're engaging in something physical, such as running a marathon, your endurance will be increased along with your blood flow, and your breathing and heart rate will speed up so you can maximise your body's energy.

In each of these situations, the release of the vagal brake speeds up your physiology, giving you access to the resources you need to achieve your goal – even if that goal is outside of your comfort zone. And once that particular situation is over and your survival brain determines that you're 'safe' again, that vagal brake will be reactivated via the vagus nerve – slowing your heart rate down, making your breath fuller and returning you to a calmer, more connected state. As this happens, you might also feel your jaw soften or notice your thoughts slowing down. The re-engaging of this vagal brake is that big sigh of relief we often hear about. It's not just a saying, it's a real thing proven by science.

For mammals, including humans, this ability to self-regulate and get out of survival mode and into a state that supports cooperative behaviour is essential to survival. In a crisis, we pick up on danger cues from our environment as well as those around us, and shift into a survival state *together*, matching the energy of the moment and each other – allowing us to work cooperatively together for a common goal in the moment, and collectively come back to a calm, balanced state once a threat has passed.

Jenny and Selena's story: Stress and the vagal brake

One of the most important facets of the heart–brain connection – and the engagement or disengagement of the vagal brake – is the role of stress. Jenny and Selena provide a perfect example.

Jenny and Selena are middle-aged sisters who are close in age. They have a great relationship, share similar hobbies and are both outgoing, relaxed and social. Though they live in different cities, they speak regularly and support each other.

When the COVID-19 pandemic struck, both sisters were

anxious. Jenny was living alone, and Selena was living with her wife, Julia, who was immunocompromised. Initially, Selena wasn't overly worried about Julia. Despite her condition, she'd always been relatively healthy, and the two of them were taking extreme precautions to avoid becoming sick. All of them watched the daily news, quarantined, washed their hands incessantly and wore masks in public. Both sisters felt their stress levels rising as the days passed, and they worried about their loved ones. As the months wore on, both Jenny and Selena struggled with worsening anxiety and experienced shallow breathing and feelings of panic.

Despite all her precautions, Selena's wife Julia contracted the virus and was hospitalised, and in the months that followed, Selena came to the hospital as much as she was allowed. In the interim, she watched the news and tried to distract herself while remaining quarantined. Already anxious, Selena found the stress of Julia's illness almost unbearable. For the first time in her life, she started having panic attacks. Her heart would race even when she was sitting still, and she would lie wide awake almost every night.

The rapid pace of Selena's heart communicated danger signals to her brain, so initially, she shifted into a hotter sympathetic state that helped her to remain vigilant and stay actively involved with her wife's care. As Julia remained in hospital, however, Selena's emotional state started to change, and she found herself oscillating between the heat of panic and the cold of shutdown. On the few occasions she was allowed to visit the hospital and talk to the doctors about her wife's rapidly deteriorating condition, her emotions would start to spiral. Once safely back at home, she'd lie on her bed feeling completely disconnected from reality, numb and alone.

Selena was terrified and frightened, and gradually these emotions shifted her into the cold dorsal vagal state of freeze. She spent most days unable to take action or make a decision, despite the rising panic she felt inside. Three months after being hospitalised, Julia died, and Selena slipped into a deep depression. Most days, she couldn't bring herself to get out of bed, let alone do simple tasks. When she was able to get herself up and run an errand, she felt faint or weak.

By the time Jenny could visit Selena, her sister was a shell of her former self. Selena spent most of her time shut away in her room saying that she felt out of her body and numb to everything. Selena's experience of living in an anxious state, coupled with the sudden trauma of losing her wife, had changed her set point. Her inner thermostat had been turned all the way down, putting her in a cold, frozen state of immobilisation. Her new normal was apathy, exhaustion, depression and dissociation.

Jenny's baseline had shifted, too, but in the opposite direction. Since the start of the pandemic, she'd been existing in the heat of the sympathetic state – constantly fearful and anxious. Julia's death had turned up the heat to such a degree that the ping of a news alert on her phone could make her palms sweaty. Officially, the worst of the pandemic was over, but the way Jenny interacted with people had fundamentally changed. She'd gone from being extroverted and social to someone who felt anxious in groups. Even socialising with a few friends was too much for her.

Throughout the pandemic, Jenny's body had been sending signals of danger to her brain. Those signals, coupled with worries about her sister's declining mental health, had activated stress responses in Jenny's survival brain. With each threat her brain perceived, she shifted higher into that hotter sympathetic state. Her vagal brake was released more and more, causing her blood pressure to go up and flooding her with mobilising energy that fuelled her anxiety.

In some ways, this was good – even necessary. Initially, it kept Jenny safe and gave her the energy and courage to show up for her sister, despite her fears of travelling and exposing herself to so many people. In the long term, though, it was less beneficial.

Determined to get a handle on her feelings of anxiety and panic, Jenny visited her doctor, who prescribed her medication to lower that high blood pressure and sent her on her way. From a purely biological point of view, the medication worked. Jenny's blood pressure did come down a little. From a psychological and social perspective, however, her issues remained unsolved, because the feelings that had triggered the release of her vagal brake hadn't been addressed. She remained stuck in survival mode.

Jenny and Selena's story highlights the inextricable connection between our nervous systems and our physical and psychological health. Exposure to chronic stressors and trauma forces us outside our window of tolerance and keeps us there for so long that everyday life starts to feel unbearable. People who struggle with chronic depression, burnout, irritability and even anger find themselves in similar patterns, and this gives us a glimpse of how our brain impacts our heart, and vice versa.

Both women could benefit from training with resources to help them connect with their body and environment, as this might help them move back into their respective windows of tolerance, where they can then fully recover from their stress and trauma. If they can get back to that non-optimal set point, in time they'll be able to recalibrate their nervous system thermostat to a more optimal set point by using the resources and tools we'll learn about in Part Two.

Without a concerted effort by Selena and Jenny to build their autonomic awareness and re-regulate themselves, they'll be at greater risk of developing physical ailments on top of the emotional and mental stress they're already experiencing. When things are running well, our blood pressure increases as we move into the hot state, and that can help us focus, take action and do what we need to. When the stressor passes, our blood pressure returns to homeostasis. But when we face chronic or traumatic stress, there's prolonged elevation of blood pressure (i.e. hypertension). This is the allostatic load or wear and tear that accumulates in our brain–body system. Conversely, when the dorsal vagal state moves us into collapse and even shutdown, where we have a surge of immobilisation, our blood pressure and our heart rate drop and we may find it impossible to move or take action. We feel weak and faint. Exhaustion and gut issues can also creep in as our system grinds to a standstill.

Heart rate variability (HRV)

The heart's pacemaker – the sinoatrial node – determines the rate of our heartbeat and, contrary to popular belief, a healthy heart doesn't beat at a consistent rate like a metronome – it varies with our breath. When we inhale, our heartbeat speeds up because the vagal brake has relaxed its dampening effect on the heart's pacemaker. When we exhale, the beat slows because our vagal brake re-engages. This variation between the two beating rates is called heart rate variability (HRV). Simply put, HRV is the distance between our heartbeats in milliseconds (ms). There are wearable devices that track HRV, but for clinical assessments, 24-hour HRV recordings are the gold standard.

These HRV readings can provide a very useful snapshot of how efficiently our vagus nerve is working. Unlike blood pressure, however, there's no ideal HRV rate. It declines with age, varies from person to person, and changes from situation to situation, so the best way to gauge your own HRV is to monitor it over time and look for upward or downward trends in your results.

Overall, a high HRV indicates high vagal tone and a healthy vagal brake: it is also associated with more effective emotional regulation. Low HRV indicates that the vagal brake has been released to increase heart rate. This was the case for Jenny, and that higher heart rate only contributed to pushing her further into an activated state. When our HRV is chronically low, we lose the ability to relax the vagal brake a little and coast along. Instead, we release it completely and end up barrelling downhill way too fast. We can no longer shift speeds as life demands, and we move into anxiety or fight or flight any time we need to step outside our comfort zone even a little.

When this happens, we're likely to be stuck in that too hot state with elevated high blood pressure. Researchers consider low HRV an indication of future health problems, because it indicates that we're less resilient and struggle to cope with changing situations. Thankfully, however, low HRV can be addressed by improving vagal tone through the bioplasticity training we'll be exploring in Part Two.

Heart rate variability

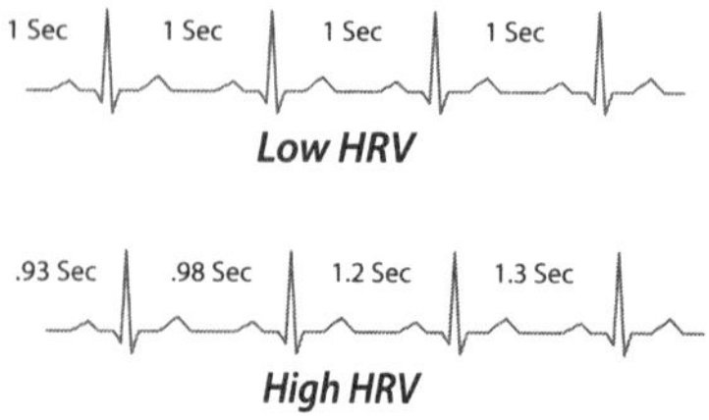

1 Sec 1 Sec 1 Sec 1 Sec

Low HRV

.93 Sec .98 Sec 1.2 Sec 1.3 Sec

High HRV

Low HRV	High HRV
'Fight or flight'	High vagal tone
Easily exhausted	Improved performance
Low adaptability	High adaptability
Decreased cognition	Improved cognition

A stronger vagal brake leads to better vagal tone

When we strengthen our vagal tone, we're better able to use this heart–brain connection to our advantage and return to regulation sooner. Ideally, our heartbeat reflects the demands of whatever is happening in our current reality – this is called *vagal efficiency*. If we're running for cover during a tornado and our heart's pounding to get oxygenated blood to our muscles so we can quickly take action, this matches the urgency of the life-or-death situation we're in – and that's vagal efficiency.

But if we notice that our heart pounds just as intensely when another driver takes the parking spot we've been waiting for, that's not good because it doesn't match the physical demands of the situation. Sure, we might feel angry (even furious), but having such a powerful physical reaction is disproportionate given there's no threat to our safety or life. If you can consciously engage the vagal brake in the moment (which you'll learn to do in Chapter 9), you'll be able to bring your heart rate down, increase your HRV and likely calm those fiery emotions in the process.

Similarly, if you're hosting a celebration dinner for a friend but feeling flat, shut down or disconnected, consciously up-regulating your nervous system is a great way of accessing more energy to meet the social requirements of that moment. The breathing exercise on page 279 is a simple tool you can use to do exactly this. The more skilled we get at deploying our vagal brake and adjusting our arousal levels to match whatever is in front of us, the better we can handle any situation life throws at us. We become more resilient and can perform better and succeed under pressure. We even have the capacity to reach peak performance.

For an athlete, peak performance might look like staying calm while harnessing maximum physical energy and focus during competition. In everyday life, peak performance might look like rising to a challenge – such as having a difficult conversation, nailing a job interview or acting quickly and efficiently in a true emergency.

Without a healthy vagal brake, we can't shift into and out of our nervous states as easily, so chronic or traumatic stress is more likely to leave us outside our window of tolerance. Too much time in this zone can either lead to hypertension (high blood pressure) or low HRV, which are common in people with persistent pain and gut disorders.

The human gut

If you're confident that you understand the anatomy of the human gut, you can skip this box, but if you can never quite remember where exactly things are and what they do, here's a quick refresher.

When we put food in our mouth, the first stage of digestion occurs as we mix it with our saliva, which starts to break down the starch.

When we swallow, our food moves into the *oesophagus* through a valve called the upper *oesophageal sphincter* that closes behind it. The food then passes through a second valve, the lower oesophageal sphincter, which also closes again immediately.

In the *stomach*, the food is mixed with hydrochloric acid and other secretions and churned for 90 minutes to four hours. The acid, along with enzymes, starts disassembling proteins into their component amino acids.

When the partially digested food reaches an appropriate consistency, the stomach intermittently releases it into the *small intestine* via a valve called the *pyloric sphincter*. Very little food has been absorbed into the bloodstream at this point. Also often referred to as the small bowel, the small intestine is very long and highly folded.

The partially digested food is mixed with bile, which has been made in the liver and stored in the gallbladder, entering the intestine via the bile duct. The bile starts breaking down fats, and enzymes entering from the pancreas digest them still further. The pancreas also sends enzymes that keep breaking down carbohydrates and proteins, while the intestine itself also adds some digestive enzymes to the mix.

In the next part of the small intestine, 90 per cent of nutrient absorption occurs. Nutrients of every kind are transported into the bloodstream and taken to cells throughout the body. The remaining food – which is now largely water and indigestible fibre – slows as it reaches the last part of the small intestine. This is where the *gut microbiota* – our population of gut microorganisms – starts to increase. A little more absorption occurs, and the food then moves into the large intestine, also often called the large bowel.

The colon, the longest part of the *large intestine* is an important part of the digestion process. The digested food can take as long as 30 hours to move along it. The *colon* absorbs excess water from the digested food to transform it into stools, but it's also where the gut microbiota is at its most populous. Here, bacteria feed on the fibre we've been unable to digest.

The *rectum* acts as an assembly point for faeces, which builds up until the next bowel movement through the *anus*. And thus, 24–60 hours after we ate it, the journey of our food is complete.

Human digestive system

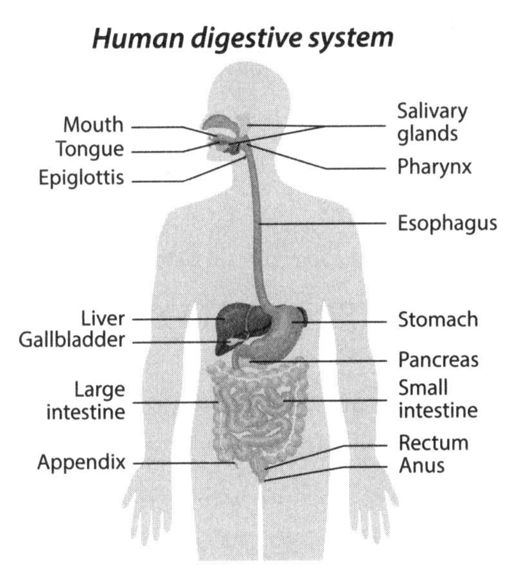

The gut-brain axis

At the beginning of the book, we explored how feelings of nervousness or worry often show up as sensations in our belly. We might have butterflies, feel nauseous or even need to run for the bathroom. That's because the gut, like the heart, also has distinctive features that facilitate constant two-way communication with the brain.

The 600 million neurons governing the function of the gastrointestinal tract make up the enteric nervous system, a mesh-like network often nicknamed the *second brain*. These neurons are responsible for sending appetite and hunger cues to the actual brain. Predominantly, these cues travel via the vagus nerve, but appetite and hunger messages also travel as hormonal signals via the bloodstream. How much food we eat is influenced by our sensitivity to these satiety signals as well as interoceptive signals, the social situation we're in and any stressors.

The neural circuits of this enteric nervous system control blood flow, mucus secretions and even regulate immune and endocrine (hormone system) functions. This means the gut can work somewhat independently of the brain and doesn't have to involve it in the messy daily grind of digestion and excretion – hence, the nickname second brain.

Another one of the gut's distinctive features are the neuropod cells, special sensory cells that line the stomach and intestines. These gather information from the gut wall – for instance, the stretch when our stomach is full or the pressure we might feel if there's something pressing into our gut – and fire those messages up to the brain via both the vagus nerve and hormonal signals. Once the brain has processed that information, it replies with brain-down signals (see pages 139–40 for tools to strengthen the gut–brain axis).

The vagus nerve plays an important role in helping the sympathetic, endocrine, immune, enteric nervous systems and gut microbiota work together and communicate with the brain to maintain that all-important state of homeostasis. But it also helps connect the emotional and cognitive areas of our brain with gut health. The brain also responds to stimuli from the gut by activating specific systems and organs.

Just as the gut can signal feelings of appetite and satiety to the brain, the brain can communicate cues of digestion to the gut. In the gastrointestinal tract, a process known as peristalsis – where muscles contract and relax to create movement – lets food pass through the system. The vagus nerve plays a key role in this. After moving food along the oesophagus, it allows for it to be swallowed. And when the ventral branch of the vagus nerve relaxes oesophageal sphincters – the valves between the oesophagus and stomach – food passes into the stomach.

This vagal branch also relaxes the pyloric sphincter – the valve between the stomach and intestines – so food can pass into the intestines. Promising new research shows that vagus nerve stimulation may improve gastric emptying of the stomach by increasing the opening of the pyloric sphincter.

Our gut microbiota

Of the trillions of microbes (bacteria, viruses and fungi) that exist peacefully inside us, the majority live in our intestines. They are small but mighty, and even the tiniest microbe plays a role in our overall wellbeing. Collectively, these microorganisms are known as our *gut microbiota*, and in the past decade research into the microbiota has grown exponentially as the vitally important role it plays in so many systems, including our immune system and our emotional and mental wellbeing, has come into focus.

These gut microorganisms perform a variety of essential tasks, including warding off illness. They also produce neurotransmitters (chemicals such as serotonin, dopamine and GABA) that transmit messages to the brain, influencing our brain chemistry through various pathways, including the vagus nerve. These microbes are so essential to the smooth running of our body that the gut microbiota has been labelled a supporting organ.

Much like our nervous system, our microbiota – particularly the one within our gut – is unique to us. Though the basic composition of our microbiota is fairly solidified by the age of two, it continues to change throughout our lives, since it's a product of several biopsychosocial factors such as our genetic predisposition, environment, sleep patterns, exercise and the medications we take. It's also heavily impacted by what we eat, as some diets are richer in beneficial bacteria (probiotics) and in foods that feed our gut microbiota and keep it flourishing and diverse (prebiotics). We'll explore diet and the microbiota in more detail in Chapter 11.

As with the other organs in the body, dysregulation in the gut can cause big changes in the conditions of our digestive tract. Chronic stress can alter the pH balance within the gut and also influence motility and mucus secretions, and these changes affect the health of our microbiota.

The brain–gut–microbiota axis is just one of the ways our microbiota influences our health. As with all other systems, the communication flows both ways. Just as microbes can impact our health and behaviour, our psychological states can alter our gut health. This is why changes in this axis are often associated with gastrointestinal disorders, depression, anxiety and decreased cognitive abilities.

When we don't take care of our gut health or neglect the connection between the brain and gut, our gut microbiota can become imbalanced. This is known as gut dysbiosis, and it can lead to changes in the compounds released by the microbiota, which can cause adverse immune responses. Dysbiosis can also affect how the vagus nerve signals the brain.

Sleep, lack of exercise, poor diet and many other factors can cause dysbiosis and trigger an immune response such as inflammation, which is a significant contributor to mental health disorders such as anxiety and depression, and is linked to gastrointestinal disorders such as IBS and inflammatory bowel disease (IBD).

We can imagine the microbes in our gut as seeds in soil. The key to regulation is enhancing the soil to create a healthier gut and modulate that gut–brain axis. Just as we can regulate ourselves using the other systems in the body, we can rebalance and regulate our gut microbiota through thoughtful autonomic awareness and everyday lifestyle changes such as those in Chapter 11.

The immune system and the gut

Previously, it was believed that the gut only emitted local immune responses to tackle issues in that system – e.g. maintenance and repair of gut tissue – but that isn't the case. It's now widely recognised that our gut microbiota affects the body's *entire* immune system. As much as 70–80 per cent of our immune cells occur in the gut. The gut microbiota is essential in shaping the development of our immunity and, in turn, the immune system shapes the gut microbiota. The immune system has evolved a symbiotic relationship with the microbes in our gut, and the gut microbiota thus plays a fundamental role in immune function.

The vagus nerve helps keep this immune system in check by stimulating the release of the neurotransmitter acetylcholine, which is used throughout the entire body, including the enteric nervous system. Acetylcholine slows the heart after stress and helps to keep rogue immune cells in check, which means it stops the immune system from overreacting to perceived threats, as it might with allergies and hypersensitivities, and even autoimmune conditions such as rheumatoid arthritis.

But if we're in a dysregulated state and our vagal tone has decreased, our immune system may fail to function properly and become either hyper- or hyporeactive. If we're chronically anxious and in a state of panic, or in complete shutdown and experiencing depression, our antibodies (proteins that protect you when an unwanted substance enters your body) may not be able to detect foreign microbes as effectively, and our immune system won't be summoned to fight those pathogens off quickly enough. This is why a period of chronic stress often leads to a period of sickness or illness. If dysregulation causes our immune system to become overactive, we might experience skin conditions and inflammation. We may also become more susceptible to disease.

Stress and dysregulated eating

Dysregulated eating and stress can function on a feedback loop just like all our other systems. If you've ever experienced stress, you probably know a thing or two about dysregulated eating. Anyone who's experienced a stressful day at work will probably be able to relate to this inability to notice hunger cues. Running around, completing tasks and answering emails prevents many of us from noticing our bodily signals. Later, when we realise we haven't eaten, we might say we didn't have enough time to eat, but that's not the whole story. It's more likely our brain didn't note our hunger cues while we were in that state of hyperarousal.

When we're chronically stressed, levels of the hunger and fullness hormones ghrelin and leptin are thrown off balance. We produce *more* ghrelin, which makes us crave foods that are high in sugar and fat, but *less* leptin, which regulates appetite.

When our body chemistry changes in this way, we also experience changes in interoception. It gets harder for the body to recognise satiety and hunger. By consuming the calorie-rich types of food that ghrelin makes us crave, we get a hit of the feel-good hormone dopamine, which gives us a momentary break from feeling anxious. But this is an artificial form of self-regulation, and since it fails to address the real underlying issue of a dysregulated nervous system, it can't shift us back inside our window of tolerance.

Comfort food doesn't comfort in the long term

Believe me, I'm not here to judge anyone's eating habits – particularly during moments of chronic stress or dysregulation. We've all reached for the hot chips or tub of ice cream after a bad day. That said, it's important for us to be very aware that using food as a resource to cope with stress isn't a sustainable or healthy strategy in the long term.

Eating the calorie-rich, high-fat, high-sugar foods we crave when dysregulated is a coping mechanism that ensures this dysregulated eating pattern persists. And if we experience the feelings of shame that often accompany these eating patterns, our nervous system dysregulation will actually get worse and feed this cycle.

Brain-down methods of controlling these eating patterns, such as goal setting or using willpower, might work occasionally, but if our body-up signals are overwhelming – as they tend to be when we're dysregulated, they'll likely win out in the end.

We're eating to cope with our feelings and satisfy our true need, which is to feel safe and regulated. That's why regulating our nervous system is the best way to deal with this stress eating in the long term. By engaging the vagus nerve to calm our systems, we can bring ourselves back within our window of tolerance, and as our hormone levels stabilise, it will become easier to return to our normal patterns of eating (see the exercise on pages 139–40).

Damien's story: Why a regulated gut matters

Damien was a healthy, adventurous 36-year-old who loved his job. He'd worked at the same accounting firm since graduating from university a decade earlier. He earned a good wage, and had a comfortable lifestyle and a thriving social network. He'd met most of his closest friends through his job, so it was a big part of his identity.

A few months into the recession, his company laid off 30 per cent of its staff, including Damien and several of his friends. He was devastated about losing his job, and felt very anxious for the first time in his life. He hadn't anticipated being let go, and he didn't have as much money tucked away for emergencies as he would have liked. The redundancy package his firm had given him would last for a few months, but beyond that he wasn't sure how he'd be able to pay his mortgage and meet his student loan repayments. He began looking for a new job immediately, but his firm wasn't the only one making cutbacks. The job market was crowded, and roles for accountants were thin on the ground.

In an effort to save as much money as he could, Damien swapped nights out with mates for weekends alone playing video games or watching movies. Reluctantly, he cancelled his gym membership as well as the skiing trip he'd booked with his brother. Around this time, Damien started experiencing discomfort in his gut, which was unusual for him. Since he hadn't changed his diet and had no history of gut issues or pain, he began paying more attention to his daily routine and noticed that his bowel movements were far less regular. Unsure of why this would be, he resolved to drink more water and assumed it probably had to do with him not eating as much as he had before losing his job. It wasn't that he was avoiding food; he just didn't feel that hungry most of the time.

When one of his friends got engaged, Damien and his friends made plans to have a rare night out. He couldn't wait to see everyone, but shortly after arriving at the pub he started feeling bloated – even nauseated. He tried ignoring those feelings, but they persisted. *I don't want to throw up in front of my mates,* he thought as he scanned the room for a bathroom. Though he tried to keep up with the conversations at the table, Damien couldn't concentrate because of his thoughts. He worried that something was seriously wrong with him. What if he'd contracted a virus? What if he got so sick that he couldn't look for a job for the next month?

Distracted by his racing thoughts and the painful spasms in his gut, Damien excused himself and found a bathroom. To his disappointment, he didn't have a bowel movement, but he did notice that his body relaxed a little. He re-joined the group, but when he couldn't stop worrying about what was wrong with him, he made an excuse and headed home. Once back at the apartment, he felt okay, and assumed he must have eaten something at the pub that didn't agree with him.

When Damien's stomach began churning on the way to meet a friend at a restaurant the next week, he had a sense of déjà vu. He felt bloated and sick again within minutes of arriving, and though he managed to stay a little longer this time, it still ruined his evening. The next day, he booked an urgent appointment with his doctor, who suspected that he had heartburn or maybe IBS. Unable to pinpoint a precise cause, the doctor recommended Damien pick up a pack of antacids on his way home.

At this point, Damien had been out of work for nearly three months, and the financial stresses of unemployment, along with a drastically reduced social life, had weakened his immune system. The ongoing anxiety and worries about his future had shifted his nervous system into a too hot state, and those messages of danger had reached his gut, which had obediently responded to the imminent 'threat' by switching to survival mode. His gut motility had slowed right down and his hunger cues had been dulled. Mucosal secretions in his gut were reduced along with stomach emptying, and blood flow to the gut was diverted to his limbs.

This chronic stress had no doubt affected Damien's gut microbiota, too. Changes in peristalsis likely caused his constipation, and that, paired with his disordered eating, meant that his microbiota wasn't receiving the nutrients it needed to function properly. Over time, his constipation, pain and bloating were the interoceptive cues that alerted his built-in threat detection system. After his brain received the message that something was wrong, it determined (neurocepted) that this assumption was correct, and then triggered stress responses that fuelled even more racing thoughts, which in turn triggered a greater stress response.

Damien's dysregulated eating patterns were a classic symptom of chronic stress, since changes in interoception can cause internal signals to register as either 'too quiet' or 'too loud'. His extended period in that hotter state of sympathetic activation outside his window of tolerance meant he wasn't noticing cues of hunger, leaving him without any real interest in food. When our hunger cues become too quiet to interocept, we might skip meals without realising and find ourselves feeling agitated or even lightheaded. External cues, such as seeing other people eat their lunch, or noticing that it's lunch time might remind us that we need to eat, but we won't necessarily feel hungry.

On the other hand, when our signals are too loud we might become *overly* sensitive to them, and even feel anxious or overwhelmed by signals of hunger. This might cause us to overeat. A positive takeaway from this is that we have the ability to partner with this system and make our interoception more accurate.

Had Damien's difficult year shifted him into the cold or dorsal vagal state, his symptoms could have been very different. In a collapsed state, his survival brain would have communicated to his gut via the vagus to empty his bowels, and instead of feeling constipated, he might have experienced bouts of diarrhoea. From a primal point of view, expelling the contents of our intestines could be a useful response, since shedding excess weight would make us a fraction lighter and allow us to move faster and escape.

Without intervention, the change in the feedback loop between Damien's body and brain, moving away from homeostasis, is an example of bioplasticity. His brain and gut would become more sensitive to stress, and his threshold for pain or anxiety would decrease. His survival brain might 'learn' to respond to similar situations in the future with the same symptoms of anxiety and decreased gut motility.

That means that even once all of these stresses were behind him, Damien could find himself feeling sick to his stomach on a night out with friends, without any apparent stimulus. He might begin to feel anxious and worried about becoming sick in public or having to find a bathroom, or even about his pain worsening.

Accurate interoception and the appropriate deployment of the right resources, can ensure we don't experience this long-term response. Of course, this doesn't mean that Damien's pain should be dismissed. It is real pain and should be viewed as part of a bigger puzzle. Increasing vagal tone and improving his interoceptive accuracy would help Damien uncouple the thoughts and emotions from his bodily signals, which amplify his symptoms and feed his dysregulation.

The road back to regulation

Damien's story helps us envisage the gut–brain connection in action, but looking at his physical pain and other symptoms in isolation doesn't give us the full picture. For that, we need to take a biopsychosocial approach and consider the other factors playing into his health challenges – namely, his genetic predisposition, his mental state before these episodes, his access to support, his employment and the health of his social relationships. All of these variables can impact our set point and influence this kind of dysregulation.

Research shows that gastrointestinal disorders and nervous

system dysregulation often go hand in hand, and that the rate of IBS and gastrointestinal disorders is four times higher in people with anxiety than those without it. The rate of anxiety is also five times higher in people with IBS than in those without this condition. Had Damien's doctor approached his case from a biopsychosocial perspective and asked more questions about his current circumstances, emotional wellbeing and anxiety levels, Damien may have been able to get closer to the real cause of his distress sooner.

Similarly, if Damien had more autonomic awareness and knowledge of interoceptive exercises such as the one on pages 139–40, he might have managed to bring his nervous system back within his window of tolerance before slipping into dysregulation. In a calmer state, his brain would have been better able to receive the hunger cues from his gut and interpret them accurately, prompting him to eat and likely heading off some of the issues he ended up facing.

Unfortunately, in a perfect (but unfortunate) example of the gut–brain feedback loop in action, Damien's psychological health was reflected in his organ function, and vice versa. If he'd remained outside his window of tolerance for much longer, he might have seen a long-term shift in his immunity and a lowered ability to fight off viruses and infections.

To bring himself back to regulation, Damien built his autonomic awareness by practising regular body-up interoception training so he could better recognise what was really going on in his body. This meant regularly tuning in to his sensations in order to identify hunger cues, and noticing how eating different foods made him feel, mentally and physically. By becoming aware of the sensations in his gut and paying attention to how it responded to different stimuli, as well as using resources to shift out of the too hot state when he worried about his work, he strengthened his vagal tone and got better at noticing when he was shifting outside his window of tolerance. This allowed him to regulate himself before things got too out of hand.

Though he didn't land a permanent job right away, Damien did secure a year-long contract that took some of the financial pressure off. Though the prospect of future unemployment still worried him, by using breathing resources to calm himself and going swimming a few times each week, he was better able to discharge that anxious energy and engage the logical part of his thinking brain, which knew that he would find another job as long as he kept looking.

The breathing exercises and discharging of excess energy through gentle exercise sent body-up signals to his survival brain that there wasn't any danger. In response, his brain told his organs (in this case, his gut) that it was okay to relax and motility was restored once he re-entered his window of tolerance. Studies have indicated that engaging this kind of body-up training where we change the signals being sent from the body to the brain, may reduce gut symptoms such as abdominal pain, bloating and nausea by as much as 70 per cent in some people with IBS. This was certainly Damien's experience. After three months of consistent conscious nervous system work, he reported that he was no longer experiencing the symptoms and that he felt better than he had in a long time.

Strengthening his vagal tone allowed Damien to modulate his gut–brain axis when necessary, and meant he could finally address the real root of the issue: his dysregulated nervous system. As we've explored, this work is well worth doing, since increased awareness of the gut–brain connection improves function in several important areas:

- gut motility
- peristalsis
- gut secretions
- stomach emptying
- the immune system.

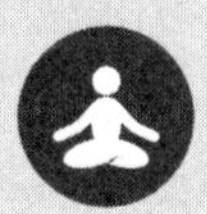

Exercise: The gut-brain axis and dysregulation

In your notebook or journal, reflect on the following questions. Your responses may indicate physiological changes that are symptomatic of an extended period of dysregulation.

- Do you tend to notice feelings of satiety and hunger easily, or is it difficult?
- Do you often go for large periods of time without eating and not realise it?
- Do you often feel drawn to calorie-rich foods?
- If you're feeling stressed, do you gravitate toward a specific type of food?
- Do you ever experience racing thoughts in response to gut pain or sickness that drive dysregulation?
- When gut sensations arise, do you notice an autonomic response: for example, fear and worry, along with ruminating thoughts about what you ate? Or do you feel shutdown, hopelessness and thoughts like *This will never get better*?
- Do you struggle with IBS, IBD or other gut disorders?

- Do you find that you frequently experience constipation or diarrhoea? Or have they occurred only at specific times in your life?
- Do you experience frequent gut pain? Bloating?
- Do you recognise any patterns between your symptoms and your nervous system thermostat?

Fascia and the nervous system

The fibrous web of tissue that surrounds our muscles, blood vessels and nerves, connecting them to each other, is called *fascia*. Fascia extends into every structure and system in the body and has approximately 250 million nerve endings, making it one of the largest sensory organs in the body. This means that fascia is an important part of the brain–body system, and carries a lot of vital information to and from the brain. Despite this, many people don't know what it is or why it's important.

While fascia holds our organs and other structures in place, it also stretches and slides smoothly to allow us freedom of movement. We have several different types of fascia in superficial layers just under the skin as well as deeper layers that wrap around our bones, muscles and organs. The layer of superficial fascia that sits below the skin shares the same receptors as the skin. The deep fascia that wraps around our organs, such as our heart, lungs and digestive system, are rich in autonomic nervous system nerves, making this an important layer for interoception. It influences the body's ability to transmit hormones through the body – such as adrenaline when it's in the hot state and oxytocin (the hormone of attachment and bonding) when it's in the just-right state – as well as neurotransmitters such as serotonin, dopamine, GABA and acetylcholine. Deep fascia also plays a role in proprioception– the sixth sense that tells us where our body is in space at any given time.

While by nature, fascia expands and contracts in line with the physical movements of everyday life, when we experience a physical injury or emotional trauma – for example, when we go into shock and collapse or freeze – our movement tends to become restricted. This ensures our survival in the moment, but with ongoing patterns of collapse and freeze, and dissociation from our body, this lack of movement, combined with emotional stress, physical injury and historical trauma, is thought to potentially impact fascia, but more research is needed for us to say for sure how stress and trauma affects it.

Research indicates that people who have experienced long-term hyperarousal or hyperarousal as a result of childhood trauma often express higher sensitivity for pain.

Fascia and persistent pain

The brain is constantly evaluating messages coming from the sensory nerve endings (nociceptors) embedded in the skin and fascia, because these are the first organs to detect any stimuli from damaged or potentially damaged tissue. If, after considering past experiences, thoughts and environmental cues, the brain concludes that there's real physical danger, it will trigger a pain sensation.

Pain is a protective mechanism created by the brain to stop us from damaging ourselves further, and this is an incredible thing. In acute injury situations, this pain cue is appropriate, but if the brain gets stuck in this protective state, then these nociceptors can become more sensitive than before, making us more susceptible to pain, anxiety, depression and a host of other ailments.

How we experience pain is entirely individual. Pain, like trauma, is highly subjective and a sensation that's perceived as painful by one person may be perceived as uncomfortable, not painful, or even pleasant to another. For example, two people may go for a massage with the same therapist and one may find the pressure painful and too strong, while another person may find it relieving and incredibly relaxing.

Just like we have neuroception as an inner threat detection system that predicts what state we move into, the threat value of pain information is important as well – the context matters. And our past experience colours how we experience pain too. Our emotions can make the pain experience more unpleasant, and our thoughts, attention, expectations and reappraisal can decrease or increase how we experience pain. This is why understanding your brain–body system can have a direct impact on physical pain and nervous system activation.

There is no one specific brain area dedicated to pain. It exists in networks through various regions in the brain. This is also true for emotions. These are known as the pain network and the interoceptive network, respectively (see pages 148–51). The pain network is found within the interoceptive network.

Interoceptive and pain signals from your body travel up towards the brainstem along the same afferent pathways (the spinal cord and vagus nerve), then on to the rest of the brain. As your body talks to your brain, there is 'crosstalk' among neurons, and they impact each other along the way. You might imagine them as different planes on their way to the same airports and the pilots are radioing each other about their location and when they'll land. Because of this network, planes that fly in from our organs, muscles and joints, plus the planes involved in our thoughts, beliefs and expectations, will determine how we experience both our emotions and pain.

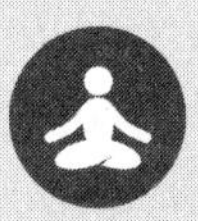

Exercise: Visualise your fascia

To strengthen your understanding of the connection between fascia and ongoing pain, clench a fist while you read this passage. Picture every muscle in your fingers and arms tightening, which occurs (unconsciously) when our nervous system switches into the sympathetic state of fight-or-flight and there's more 'bracing'. This is what happens to our fascia when we're on guard and ready to take on a threat or flee. It's easy to see how this type of tightening throughout your entire body for months or even years could cause pain and other issues.

Let's try something different. Let your hand go completely limp and visualise this limpness extending to every muscle in your body. Everything from your shoulders to your jaw slackens completely. Essentially, this is what happens to fascia when you're in that cold dorsal vagal state. Now think about how difficult it would be to go about your daily life – run errands, meet friends, pick up kids from school – while experiencing this floppy and collapsed dorsal vagal state.

The importance of working with our fascia

To feel our best, we need to make restoring our relationship with our body a priority. Knowing where our body is in space helps bring us back to regulation. Being able to unlock our body from rigidity when we're frozen or bracing, or reintroduce structure when we're collapsed can also bring us back to regulation. When we work with our fascia, we access a doorway to our entire autonomic nervous system, and this helps us physically and mentally.

We can wake up the connection between the autonomic nervous system and the fascia, and influence our brain–body system in a positive way, by using bioplasticity resources that target the fascia and focusing our attention on our muscles, organs and heartbeats (proprioception + interoception). By breathing deeply, stretching, employing pressure and touch to different sensory receptors throughout our body and using resources like the ones we cover in Chapters 11 and 12, we can reinstate and strengthen this connection between our mind and body. First, though, it helps to understand how our brain *perceives* our body.

Map of the brain's sensory cortex

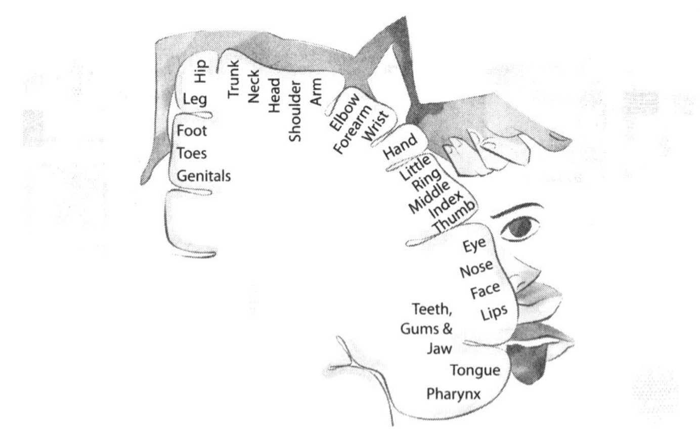

I know this diagram looks funny, but it gives us a pretty good idea how the brain 'maps' individual body parts. It uses this map to let us know where our body is in space. This particular image shows a cross-section of the brain's mapping from the top of your head down towards your ear. If you look at this illustration again, you'll notice that more sensitive areas of the body take up the most space. The lips and the tongue, for example, occupy more space in this drawing than the head and shoulders, and that's because it's easier for us to recognise sensations in these areas of our body than it is in the trunk or shoulders.

Hands, too, are drawn in a way that shows how much sensory processing information they gather for the brain, telling it exactly where our hands are and what they're doing. We can tell when they are being touched or touching something else, and our ability to move our fingers with precision means we can perform intricate tasks such as surgery or plating up Michelin-star dishes. Our life experiences continue to shape this map. For example, the representation of fingers and hands on the brain map of a violinist is likely show them taking up even more space than those of the average person. This is another example of how bioplasticity shapes us throughout our life.

Phantom limb pain, which is when we experience pain in a body part that doesn't exist, can teach us a lot about how the brain maps body parts, as well as the pain network in our brain. A leg may be missing, but the leg and its relationship to the rest of the body is still represented in that map within the brain and areas throughout brain networks. Incredibly, someone born without arms and legs can still experience phantom limb pain, which tells us that a sensory map for our limbs exists from birth. To the brain, these non-existent limbs are completely real and so is the pain from them. The pain not only feels real, but it can also get worse with stress.

Studies using brain imaging have shown that this brain map is significantly altered in cases of phantom limb pain. Not only is the map less clear, but the area representing the missing limb is less well defined, and may appear as 'smudges'. Pain from this area may also be felt in the other areas of the body, such as the face.

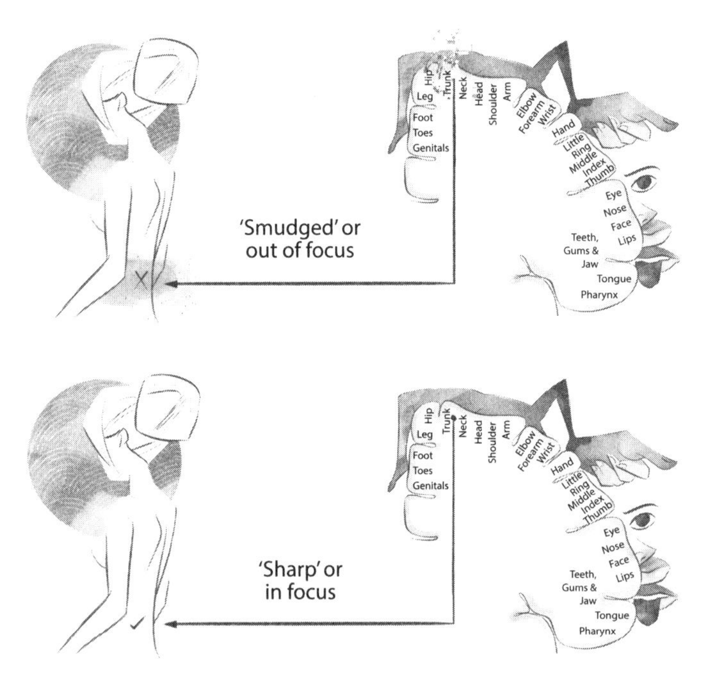

'Smudging' occurs when the body image in the brain becomes 'out of focus'. It's thought to lead to decreased body awareness (interoception). The bottom image shows the intact – 'in focus' – body schema.

This 'smudging' phenomenon also seems to be true for many people who experience persistent pain such as fibromyalgia. The technical name for this smudging is 'central sensitisation', and it can result in pain messages from the body becoming blurred and unclear, making it harder for the brain to understand which area needs protection.

Let's say you break the index finger on your left hand and have to keep it taped to your middle finger for four weeks while it heals. Over the course of those weeks, the representation of your left hand in the brain will adapt to reflect these two fingers being taped together. In the short term, this protective mechanism can be really helpful, because it will prevent you from overusing that injured finger while it heals. Ideally, once you remove that tape, your finger will be pain-free and you'll get back to using that hand normally. And after a few hours of this, your brain map will revert to the way it was before.

If, however, you experience pain in your index finger when you remove that tape and continue to restrict the movement of that finger, your brain might conclude that those two fingers need extra protection and call on neighbouring parts of the hand to help. In this scenario, that brain map won't revert to the way it was before. It may even change further if this goes on for long enough. In this case, we might begin not to be able to distinguish one finger from the other or use them with precision or independently. The pain from that one finger might even start to smudge to other areas of the hand and other body parts.

A biopsychosocial approach to treating pain

With a better understanding of how the brain changes in people with persistent pain, we have a better chance of treating that pain effectively by taking a biopsychosocial approach. Rather than hunting down the source of persistent pain as if it's an ongoing injury, it's often better to take an integrative approach – with the help of a health professional.

Sensations, whether they are overwhelming bodily signals, emotional distress, physical pain or even social pain such as rejection, involve changes to the way body-up and brain-down signals are processed, as well as changes to the interoceptive network within the brain. When the smudging effect occurs, it's often due to amplification of pain signals in the brain rather than one specific injury. Immune system responses can cause pain, and in these cases anything that calms the immune system can help. As we'll explore in Chapter 11, this includes spending time inside our window of tolerance, bolstering our gut microbiota, and getting enough exercise and sleep.

Integrating all of the body-brain systems

Years ago, when I was a physiotherapist in training, I studied textbooks of colour-coded diagrams detailing the ins and outs of each bodily system, and that knowledge served me well for many years. But it was only once I learned about the vagus nerve and the nervous system in more detail that all of these pieces finally fell into place.

For me, that was the 'a-ha' moment that brought everything together. It was as though every 2D diagram I'd studied suddenly layered on top of each other and became 3D. It was so clear to me that *all* of our systems, from our brain and gut to our fascia and nerves, slotted together into one sensitive, interconnected system. This is the essence of 'whole person' health.

Once these disparate elements had converged into one entity for me, it was impossible to go back to seeing them the way I had before. Treating issues in isolation no longer made sense when the impact of our choices, past experiences, behaviours and challenges on our health was so clear. When you see how your interoceptive network underpins so much of your physiological functioning, it becomes undeniable that whatever patterns you've learned can also be unlearned, and *that* is exciting.

Imagine that there are different airports located throughout the brain–body system.

This is where there are collections of neurons with a specific function.

For example, in the body there's the enteric nervous system in the digestive system, collectively also known as our 'second brain'.

Body-up messages (planes) that travel from the body to the brain can fly via nerves (especially the vagus nerve and spinal cord), or via hormonal or immune signals.

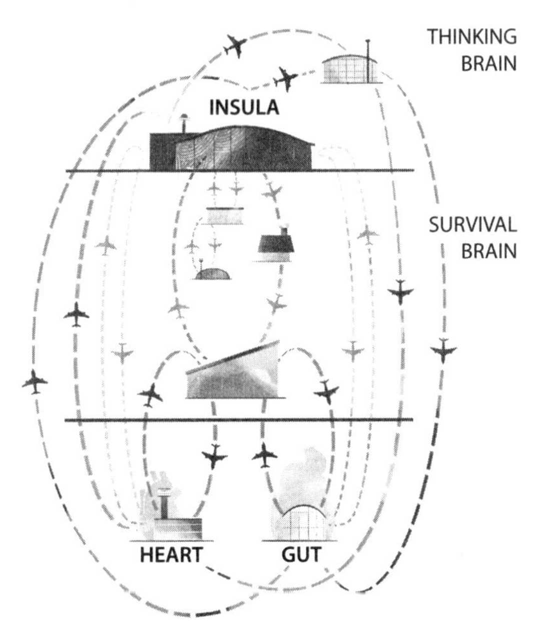

Within the brain, planes may land in 'airports' in the lower centres of the brain, such as the brainstem; together with their 'returning flight', they maintain homeostasis. Although we may be unaware of much of this information, it creates a feedback loop that maintains internal balance and stability. You might think of it like catching a flight to a city and then taking your returning flight home, returning you to your normal way of life.

Some signals from our body do reach our conscious awareness, particularly when they land at one of the biggest airports, the insula. We can think of this as like Heathrow Airport, one of the world's busiest. Not only does it have flights returning to the body, but it also has connecting flights with other airports throughout our brain that impact how we experience emotions, pain or distress.

As we can see in the diagram below, these are the most important 'airports'.

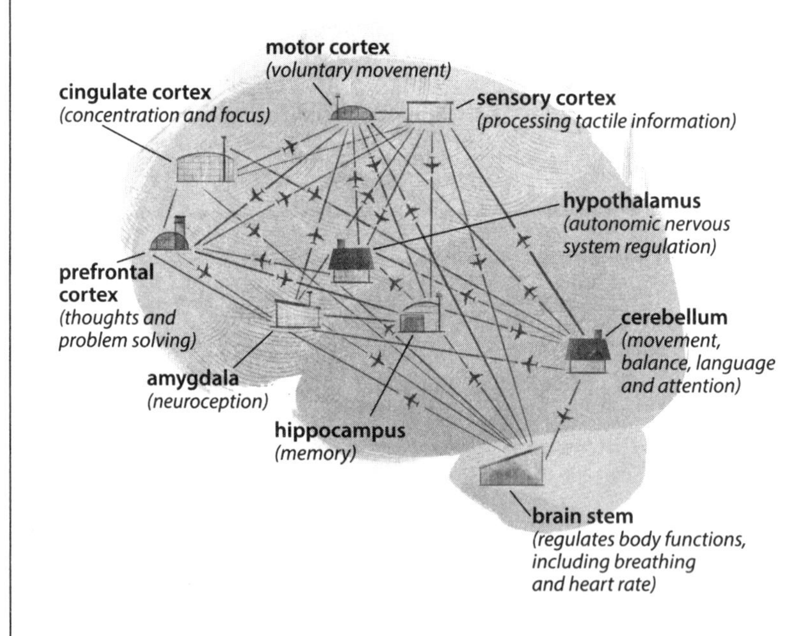

As planes fly from the insula to the frontal lobe, the thoughts we have, the language we use and our beliefs all influence where the planes go next in our body. If we feel sensations of fear and our thoughts and beliefs sound like *It's all going to fall apart*, the plane that flies back into our body may inhibit the regulating effect of the vagal brake on our heart, causing us to shift into anxiety and fight or flight.

This isn't the same as trying to control our bodily sensations via brain-down planes, with minimising thoughts like *It's not that bad*, denial like *I'm fine*, or by burying, cutting off or ignoring what's happening.

To bring brain-down regulation, we want to bring awareness to what's happening, see what state we're in and then we have an opportunity to reappraise. In doing so, we're seeing reality as it is and partnering with our nervous system. This is very different from brain-down *management* that tries to control, deny and ignore.

We also know that sensations that travel up to the brain are compared there to previous experiences and these body memories can lead us to becoming triggered. The returning flight takes exactly the same path as before because the brain predicts that this situation is exactly the same as the past.

As we practise neuroplasticity (which we will do in Part Two), we change the path of plane and the influence it has on this network. Neuroplasticity is the incredible ability of neural networks in the brain and nervous system to change through growth and reorganisation.

It's helpful for us to remind ourselves that this network that maintains homeostasis also impacts our emotions and the state of our nervous system at any given moment.

Interoceptive training for the brain–body loop

When it comes to creating change, learning must be embodied and experiential, which is why I'm going to invite you to do this interoception exercise. Once you walk through it, and as you practise it over time, you'll find you can easily use it in your everyday life in order to help improve the communication within your gut–brain axis.

Start by establishing how you're feeling at this very moment. If you suspect that you're in that hotter sympathetic state – anxious, on edge, irritable, and so on – you may want to relax back in a chair or even lie down before continuing this exercise. If you're in that more immobile, cold dorsal vagal state and feeling flat or disconnected, try sitting with an upright spine or shift into standing to up-regulate your nervous system. If you're already feeling calm and at ease, a seated position works just fine. Soften your gaze and allow your eyes to look down to the floor about one metre in front of your feet. Allow your attention and awareness to come inward.

Exercise: Tune in to your bodily signals

First make note of the preparations detailed above.

1. Start the exercise by noticing the sensations associated with your eyes, particularly the small muscles in and around them. Try to tap in to your bodily signals. Are your eyes emitting a tingling sensation? Do they feel tense? Take note of any sensations.

2. Slowly turn your attention to your mouth. What sensations do you feel on your lips? Your tongue? From there, move your attention to your jaw. Is it relaxed or tense? If you're finding it hard to tune in to any bodily signals, try opening and closing your mouth a few times to increase the sensory input.
3. Bring your attention to your throat, and try to remain curious about any sensations you notice.
4. Continue working your way slowly down your body, and direct your attention further inward as you go. Even the smallest of feelings or sensations are worth noting. This practice is all about focusing on the key areas of the body–brain loop, so as you go about this, imagine you're walking step by step through your internal system.
5. As you travel further inward, notice sensations between your breastbone (i.e. sternum, which joins your ribs on your chest), your spine, and your ribs – one by one. See if you can notice the beats of your heart. Pausing to spend some time here. If you can't notice the beats you might just notice sensations in the area of the heart.

   Then let your attention shift outwards to the chest once again, and to the shoulders and ribs, this time also noticing the muscles and fascia. Do you feel any stiffness, bracing or tension? Do you feel collapsed and heavy like it's hard to hold your head up? Note whether it's easy to connect with these areas of the body, or if you feel detached or numb from any of them.

   Your mind may drift off into stories about what each sensation means, or you may just notice that you have a general sense of feeling several emotions. Slow down a little and see if you can sift through those thoughts and emotions and identify any of them or notice the bodily signals linked to them. It may feel uncomfortable to focus on this area so intently, but stay here if you can, noticing how any of the signals shift and change.

6. Allow your focus to travel downwards, under the diaphragm. Is it easy for you to connect to bodily signals here or do they feel distant, vague or fuzzy?
7. When you reach the stomach, notice sensations. Are they easy and clear to notice or is this area numb? I invite you to place a hand right on top of your belly. As you breathe, relax into the palm of your hand, feeling the warmth of your skin against your hand. Does touching this part of your body help you connect to the bodily signals in this area?

   Again, you may notice a mix of sensations or emotions in your body. Is it possible to bring interoceptive selective attention to just the bodily signals in your gut? Thoughts and emotions might arise too – that's perfectly okay. See if you can let those fade into the background while you continue giving selective attention to your bodily signals.

   Anchor your attention to your belly and imagine that the warmth of your hand represents a sense of calmness and ease, that's spreading below the skin of your belly. Picture that warmth and steadiness travelling through your digestive tract. Bring selective attention to any feelings of warmth, calmness and ease. As you do, you're deliberately sending body-up signals to your brain.

   Again, thoughts, stories or emotions may arise, but continue directing your attention to the interoceptive signals of your belly, including the warmth, ease and calmness emanating from your hand. Stay here and notice how your nervous system may shift or change.

8. When you're ready, slowly raise your eyes and bring yourself back to the room.

 What did this interoception exercise show you?

After completing the interoception exercise, I encourage you to take a few minutes to reflect on the following questions. If you can write down your answers in a notebook or in a journal, even better. You can revisit these answers later as you get more practised, and they'll give you a good indication of how far your interoception skills have come.

- When you began this practice, how did it feel to move your attention from one area of the body to the next?
- Were some areas of the body harder to connect with than others? If so, which areas were they?
- For the parts of the body that were difficult to connect to, what feelings were present?
- What stories came up in your mind when you were focusing on those areas that were hard to connect to?
- Were there any beliefs about sensations or how your body felt, such as, 'My shoulder is broken'?
- What feelings were present in the parts of your body you connected to easily?
- As you scanned your body and brought attention to different parts, did you have any physical reactions? If so, what were they?

- Once your attention was focused on your belly, what feelings came up?
- Was it hard to connect with your belly? If so, what did that feel like?
- What thoughts came to mind as you did this exercise?
- How does your energy feel now, having completed this exercise? The same? Different? How so?

Though this exercise can be a helpful everyday tool for interoceptive training, it can also be used as a stand-alone way to build autonomic awareness in moments of dysregulation or pain. When we can pay attention to our body in this way, we become better at regulating our nervous system improving many biological processes.

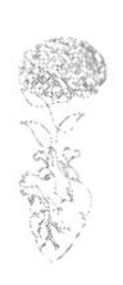

So far, much of what we've learned has centred on understanding our own nervous system and how our vagus nerve connects with some of our most vital systems and organs. Though understanding all of this and learning how to recalibrate our nervous system is absolutely essential to changing our own lives, it's equally important to recognise how our friends, colleagues or even strangers on the street can regulate us, too. Or, alternatively, they can *cause* dysregulation.

In the next chapter, we'll be exploring the third element of the biopsycho*social* model: our relationship with others. As social animals who have evolved to be part of a group, we're born hard-wired for connection with our fellow humans. And without it, we suffer.

6

The social engagement system and co-regulation

The social engagement system is primarily made up of branches of the vagus nerve that form a face–voice–heart connection, and like all the other systems we've talked about, this system is also constantly sending and receiving information that influences how safe we feel and how well we can connect with those around us. If you place one hand on your heart and your other hand on your cheek, you can envision where the social engagement system travels, along with other connections to nerves that innervate the face and middle ear. These three areas of the body communicate with each other in a constant feedback loop, and the signals in this loop also get communicated to the brain, and can either regulate us or shift us towards dysregulation.

When we're around someone who is experiencing high levels of stress activation, the tone and pitch of their voice, along with their facial expressions, gestures and body language, can excite the 'resonance circuits' in our own brain–body system. These resonance circuits biologically drive us to match the emotions of the other person. We might approach someone with the intention of connecting, but if their response isn't welcoming, our internal circuitry adapts accordingly.

This social engagement system is rooted in our primal past. Early humans needed each other to survive, and this system evolved to unconsciously gather the signals of safety or danger being transmitted in the voices, facial expressions and body language of others. These signals help us quickly decipher whether a connection or situation is safe or dangerous. This allows us to flee danger, find calm connections and ultimately survive.

Each part of the social engagement system – face, voice and heart – transmits 'warmth' through things such as the tilt of the head, tone of voice, softening of the eyes, and many more unconscious things. Warmth suggests safety, and it signals to the brain that we can approach that other person and connect with them. Lack of warmth tells us the opposite, and this is why perceived warmth is the single most important quality used in deciding how to respond to others, and how others respond to us.

This social engagement system is yet another route to building vagal tone. By using it as a tool, we can send safety or danger signals to our brain–body system. Our ability to connect, register cues of safety or threat, and even attune to others around us depends on how well our vagus nerve is functioning. Our social engagement system responds to every change in our nervous system state, and vice versa.

Co-regulation

Emotionally and psychologically, relationships with other people are essential to our wellbeing, but they're also essential from a biological point of view. We're born hardwired with this *need* for connection, so if you've been worrying that wanting friendship, love and support from others makes you a needy, co-dependent, emotional or overly sensitive person – it doesn't. In fact, feeling that you belong and having relationships where you feel truly seen and held are among the most important predictors of the quality and length of our life.

The people around you are one of the most potent influences on your nervous system, because your interactions with them impact your emotions, thoughts and physiology in ways that either nourish or deplete you. Feeling lonely or isolated can cause distress in our nervous system, and without healthy connections we shift into defensive or confrontational energy, or shut down and disconnect completely. This isn't to say you should never enjoy some alone time!

Segregation, marginalisation, lack of social support, loneliness and poverty can trigger these types of survival responses. If left unchecked, these can lead to anxiety, depression, dysregulation, cardiovascular disease, inflammation, persistent pain, compromised immune functioning and gastrointestinal disorders. Conversely, being in nourishing relationships can help shift our nervous system back to a state of safety, especially after trauma.

When we're around people we're close to and they're in a regulated state, it becomes easier for us to shift into a state of safety and belonging. In this just-right ventral vagal state, rest, recovery and repair of the brain–body system can take place. Research shows that supportive social networks can even prevent us from developing diseases. Strengthening your own relational web and being able to support another person in theirs builds healthy communities, and makes you more resilient. Wellness is not a solo act.

The power of co-regulation

When we use the safety signals others are transmitting to bring us back to balance, we call this 'co-regulation' – it's a term that describes how our nervous system changes and adapts depending on the people around us. The relationships we have with the people who care for us in infancy and childhood shape how well we can self-regulate in adulthood.

Co-regulation happens automatically when parents or caregivers attend to their child's needs in the moment. When the child cries, their carers anticipate the need being expressed by the baby and provide warmth, food, and/or physical and emotional comfort in response. When a child is distressed or dysregulated, speaking calmly and giving them affection can usually meet their need for safety and security. This goes both ways, too: the child's distress can distress the parent. This process, while it may seem instinctual, actually has a long-lasting impact on how the child will function and grow over time.

Co-regulation provides the foundations that allow other systems to thrive. In the same way a house's plumbing and electrical systems need to be built around stable floors and walls, if the emotional foundations formed in early life aren't solid, there's less stability in both the autonomic nervous system *and* the areas of the brain that govern regulation and social attachment.

Even if our first relationships in life weren't secure or healthy, we can still improve in this area through training, because not all formative co-regulation happens in childhood. Co-regulation happens every day, often with strangers and without us realising that it's happening. A smile from a stranger or an expected compliment from a neighbour can regulate us just as quickly as a disapproving glance from a co-worker can dysregulate us.

When we tune in to another person and allow our internal state to resonate and reflect their balanced state, we're co-regulating. The ability to co-regulate is one of the key functions of our social engagement system, since it's in this regulated state that we're at our healthiest, and do our best learning, creating and working.

The foundation of our ability to self-regulate begins with co-regulation.

Even if we enjoy time on our own, biologically we crave connection and want to relate to those around us. If you tend to isolate yourself in difficult times, co-regulation can help you find your way home again.

Of course, more significant relationships in our lives also have the power to regulate us and dysregulate us. Time spent with a friend can send us cues of safety and warmth and actively shape our nervous system. In turn, our perceived feelings of warmth from a good friend cause us to send cues of safety and warmth right back. Of course, the opposite is also true – a negative experience with a friend or loved one that sends cues of threat (as we'll discover), can send us into dysregulation.

Empirical research has shown how leaders and managers send strong ripples into their social environment and can have a powerful effect on other people's levels of regulation (or lack thereof). Additionally, there's a growing pool of empirical study which highlights the that well-being of leaders and managers can act as 'nerve centres' for entire teams. Through stress and emotional contagion, managers can transmit perceived stress to staff. And so organisations run the risk of instigating a 'domino effect' of stress development among their employees.

Co-regulation differs from co-dependency in that we still have a sense of ourselves. Whereas with co-dependency we may lose our interoceptive awareness and the connection with our inner world and fixate externally. We know that if we lack a connection to our inner world, our sense of self (how we're doing) will come from outside of us. With co-dependency our sense of safety comes from a source external to us.

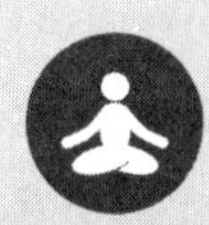

Exercise: Routes to co-regulation

In this exercise you'll be looking for your existing means of co-regulation and how you might develop more. Take out your notebook or journal and write down your responses to the following questions.

Who helps you feel a sense of belonging?

This might be a friend, relative, coach, teacher, librarian, barista, hairdresser, health professional, shop owner, mentor, classmate, gym class member, workmate or team mate.

If you don't feel you belong or don't have many connections, how can you cultivate those things?

- Reach out to new people at work to join you for lunch.

- Volunteer in your community (e.g. at an animal shelter or hospital).
- Sign up for a community art class.

When you feel like isolating and withdrawing from people, how could you make it easier to interact with other people?

- Visit a park or beach where people are.
- Go to a shopping centre.
- Work in a busy cafe or library.

Co-regulation in action

To get a better idea of what this looks like in reality, imagine yourself in the following scenarios.

You've spent all day running from one project to the next at work because there were competing deadlines, and you were so nervous about the critical feedback from your boss that you barely finished your lunch. By 5 p.m. you're exhausted and can't wait to leave the office, but instead of going straight home, you decide to meet up with a friend for a drink to catch up and chat.

Which scenario would you prefer to walk into?

- **Scenario A:** You get to the pub and spot your friend sitting at a table. She stands up and gives you a hug but avoids eye contact. You grab yourself a drink and sit down to chat, and while you're telling her about the horrendous day you've had, you notice that she lets out a few deep sighs. Her shoulders are hunched and as she isn't really responding to your stories. Her eyes are fixed on the menu on the table. You stay for an hour, but she rarely looks up from her drink, and it seems down to you to carry on the lion's share of the conversation. For the entirety of the catch-up, she's completely withdrawn.

- **Scenario B:** You walk into that same pub and see your friend waving at you with an enormous smile on her face. When you reach her, she wraps you in a big hug, makes eye contact, then sits you down – eager to hear about your 'nightmare' day. She nods as you complain about your boss and sympathises over your competing deadlines. 'Forget them!' she says, grabbing your hand. 'You're too good for that company anyway!' You both laugh.

It's pretty easy to see that scenario A will leave you feeling sullen, sad and even more stressed out, while scenario B would leave you feeling more centred, more optimistic, and more at ease and sociable. Option B for me, please!

Let's compare two more scenarios:

1. You bump into a friend you haven't seen in a long time on the street and call out as you see them. Your voice gets a bit higher as you exchange hellos and give them a hug. You make eye contact with them while smiling and talking.
2. While walking on that same street you notice a drunk stranger approaching who is shouting at passers-by. Unconsciously, you avoid eye contact with them, brace your torso and raise your shoulders.

Both examples demonstrate how quickly other people can influence our brain–body system, withdraw our vagus nerve and shift our internal systems. When we understand how others impact how we feel and act – how our physical body reacts to them, and theirs to ours – we can better rebalance ourselves, have more empathy for those around us, and even build more fulfilling relationships.

Autonomic awareness and co-regulation

The more autonomic awareness we build, the better we get at noticing how certain people affect us. As we gather that information, we can make intentional choices about who we spend time with, and what our social limits are. That's not to say you should avoid someone or cut them out of your life if they're going through a difficult time. Relationships are necessary for our physical and psychological wellbeing *and* they can be challenging and difficult. That said, if you notice that a certain relationship often lacks reciprocity and connection, or leaves you feeling overwhelmed or drained, that may be a sign to take a step back or set some limits.

When we know what our neurobiological limits are, we get better at noticing when we're reaching them. This makes it easier to take care of our nervous system because we can communicate those boundaries to others. If relationships rupture, which is a normal part of life, tapping in to our social engagement system allows us to repair those ruptures by sending those 'warm' cues to the other person, reopening the channels of communication.

The quality and quantity of our relationships is tied to how well our physical body functions and, in turn, can impact our emotional health. For this reason, possessing autonomic awareness when it comes to our social connections puts us in a better position to assess the relationships we have with people, and whether or not we have enough of the right *kinds* of connections.

Biological rudeness

One aspect of co-regulation in adulthood that doesn't get a lot of airtime is 'biological rudeness'. Coined by Dr Stephen Porges, this is when our body language and behaviour are rude – that is, they communicate coldness or indifference that may lead to a rupture in connection. Biological rudeness isn't always intentional, but it's important to highlight this behaviour because it can trigger threat responses in others and cause problems in relationships.

Let's say you're out for dinner with your romantic partner after a busy day. You've been looking forward to seeing them, especially because a disagreement you had with your best friend earlier in the week has been weighing heavily on you. You're eager to get your partner's perspective and advice on the situation.

As you begin recounting the argument, you feel vulnerable because it was your fault and you know that your friend was right to be angry with you. In the middle of your story, your partner's phone lights up with a text, and after turning it over to glance at the screen for a few seconds, your partner returns their attention to you and says, 'Go on, I'm listening.' You know they didn't look at their phone to hurt you, but this small moment or 'rupture' causes a knee-jerk response in your nervous system.

Your emotional response is instant and comes from such a deep place within you that it almost feels instinctual. That's because your nervous system doesn't care nearly as much about your partner's intentions as about their body language and behaviour. If you shift into a hotter sympathetic state when this moment occurs, your body might stiffen and you might fold your arms or respond with words of criticism, blame or even anger. If you move into a colder dorsal vagal state, you might feel a twinge of shame and think your partner doesn't consider your feelings or story important. Your posture may even collapse, or you may feel flat, and withdraw or stonewall your partner and refuse to speak.

Our nervous system state and co-regulation

Since co-regulation fundamentally impacts our brain–body system, let's take a look at how each state of our nervous system is impacted by those around us. Understanding how we receive and give cues of safety and danger (often without being aware of doing so) can help us to take a more empowered role in cultivating safe and healthy relationships. The following interactions between Jane and her mother illustrate what co-regulation and dysregulation look like in action.

Scenario 1

Jane has had a somewhat stressful week but is excited for it to finally be Saturday. Her only plan for the day is to have coffee in town with her mother, a regular activity the two of them love. When Jane arrives at the coffee shop, their respective nervous system states have a major effect how safe each of them feels, and on their interaction . . .

	Neuroception of safety	**Neuroception of threat**
Nervous system states	Jane (just right) + Her mother (just right)	Jane (just right) + Her mother (too hot)

First impressions	Jane's mother greets her at the cafe with wide-open arms and a smile. As Jane talks about her week, her mother tilts her head and listens, and nods at Jane's stories. Both Jane and her mother have their social engagement system online and it primes them for attachment.	When Jane arrives at the cafe her mother seems quite angry. She doesn't greet Jane and remains seated while avoiding eye contact. Once Jane is seated, her mother yells at her – angry that Jane missed her birthday last week.
Result	Jane neurocepts cues of safety from her mother (smiling, head tilt, listening) that allow her to anchor in the just-right state and enjoy her mother's company. They share stories and laughter, and Jane leaves the cafe feeling calm and centred. In this state, Jane has access to oxytocin and feels a warm sense of connection and belonging.	Because Jane's nervous system is calm and she's in that just-right state, she knows she can employ the social engagement system by speaking calmly while making eye contact with her mother. She nods as her mother explains why she's so upset. While apologising, Jane reaches for her mother's hand and holds it. By the end of the catch-up, her mother has calmed down and is no longer angry.
Relationship dynamics	The healthy dynamic between them showcases the high reciprocity in their relationship. There's back and forth in communication, equal attention and care given to each person and, consequently, a mutual positive reshaping of each other's nervous system.	Through reciprocity, warmth and accessing her own social engagement system, Jane was able to coax her mother's nervous system towards regulation. This isn't always possible.

Scenario 2

Jane is excited to see her mother for their coffee date. She's been so eager to tell her the big news: she was promoted at her job last week and is engaged to her long-term partner.

	Neuroception of safety	Neuroception of threat
Nervous system states	Jane (blended play state) + Her mother (just right)	Jane (blended play state) + Her mother (too hot)
First impressions	Jane runs up to her mother in the cafe and blurts out her news. The two of them hug and even jump a little, waving their hands in excitement. Jane's mum squeals with joy and can't contain her smile.	Jane runs up to her mother in the cafe and blurts out her news. To her surprise, her mother becomes incredibly angry that Jane didn't share this news with her earlier in the week. Her voice is steely and monotone, and as she crosses her arms across her chest, she accuses Jane of being deceitful.
Result	Jane neurocepts cues of safety from her mother (smiling, warmth, movement and excitement), and because she's in the play state which is the sympathetic nervous system state – mobilised, and full of energy and joyful movement. It's kept in check blended with the ventral vagal energy.	Jane's mirror neurons 'mirror' her mother's reactions before she has time to process what's happening. Jane feels reactive, and instead of feeling connected, she feels the need to protect herself. In this activated state, it's too hard for Jane to calm down enough to access her social engagement system.
Relationship dynamics	Jane was already in the state of play from her excitement about her news and her mother joined her in this state.	Jane already had more mobilising sympathetic energy and her mother's reaction felt threatening and so she shifted into fight or flight.

Scenario 3

Jane is exhausted from her week's activities. She saw friends – one who criticised her for her lack of contact that brought up quite a bit of shame. Her friend didn't invite her to another event and Jane feels isolated and excluded. Despite her exhaustion, she's agreed to see her mother for coffee because she doesn't want to miss out on catching up with her mum.

	Neuroception of safety	Neuroception of threat
Nervous system states	Jane (too cold) + Her mother (just right)	Jane (too cold) + Her mother (too cold)
First impressions	When Jane meets her mother, they sit and talk about their weeks. Jane's mother, usually always a calming presence in her life, notes that she must be extremely tired from all those social engagements. Her mother strokes Jane's hair, makes a lot of eye contact, squeezes her hand and rubs her back.	As they sit down at a table, Jane notices that her mother seems unhappy. Her arms are crossed and she's avoiding eye contact with Jane. After a few minutes of awkward silence, her mother says she's upset that Jane hasn't called her all week and she's been feeling lonely. She accuses Jane of being 'too busy' and not caring about her.
Result	Jane goes home feeling tired yet relaxed, and in need of a long nap. In her cold dorsal vagal state, Jane was able to neurocept safety from her mum's energy and body language. Consequently, she shifts towards regulation herself. Though she's not fully back within her window of tolerance by the end of their	Jane neurocepts a threat in her mother's body language and disappointed tone, and since she's already in the energy-conserving dorsal vagal state, this 'threat' causes her to spiral into shame – pushing Jane further into that colder state. She feels vulnerable, and as she shuts down emotionally,

	catch-up, Jane has shifted closer towards it and entered the blended state of 'stillness' that's associated with rest and repair. As a result, Jane feels good but sleepy.	she loses access to her social engagement system. Consequently, almost all communication is lost. Her posture shifts, and she spends the rest of their catch-up slumped in a chair with her eyes downcast. She tries listening to her mother but cannot respond.
Relationship dynamics	Jane's mother's touch and connection brought her out of the shame and feeling of not belonging that can come from the dorsal vagal state.	Jane was already feeling isolated and rejected, this, on top of her mother, spirals her further into a feeling of being disconnected with herself and others.

In each situation, the nervous system state Jane is in *before* seeing her mother impacts the way she responds to her mother's cues of safety or threat. When we can identify the nervous system state we're reacting from, we may be able to slow down and respond to others differently and even understand their reactions a bit more. Recognising our own state also helps us pinpoint what kinds of connections we need (or don't need) in that moment. The goal, of course, is to learn to employ our social engagement system in a healthy, regulated way so we can navigate cues of safety and threat with ease.

Factors that make it harder to neurocept safety cues

1. Post-traumatic stress disorder (PTSD) can impact our access to the social engagement system, and therefore our ability to regulate ourselves and others in moments of danger or even safety.
2. Neurodivergent individuals may be less able than neurotypical people to use this system to their benefit.
3. Those with auditory hypersensitivities or auditory processing difficulties and other related conditions may not find it as easy as others to neurocept safety.

In many cases, training with tools over time can improve our ability to access this system and neurocept cues. Practising these tools – especially in a one-on-one approach – while within our window of tolerance where we feel safe is a good way of 'exercising' this system.

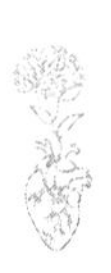

Now that you know how your nervous system works, the states it can pull you into and all the things that can influence it, you're ready for Part Two, where you will learn how to reset your nervous system by taking a more active role in the messages it's sending.

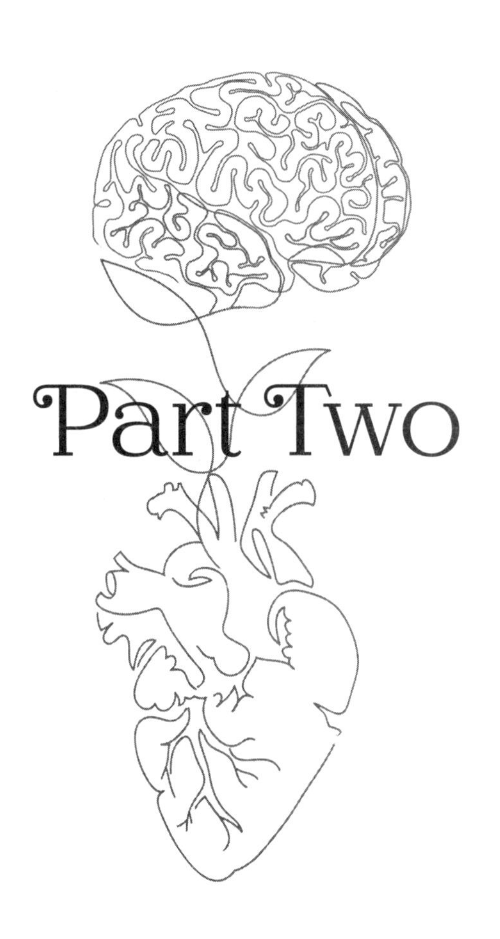

Part Two

Resetting your nervous system

The nervous system reset in practice

This part of the book is dedicated to giving you the resources you need to strengthen your interoceptive accuracy and change the way your brain neurocepts information. Each time you tune in to yourself or use a technique I've shared, you'll be retraining your body–brain system to accurately respond to the present moment. Just as this system learned to under-cope or over-cope in the past, it can relearn how to live in the now. You'll learn interoceptive awareness so you can tune in and navigate your three internal states – hot, just right and cold – and you'll learn how to partner with your nervous system to help regulate yourself.

Remember, 80 per cent of the messages whizzing around your vagus nerve, which is a major part of your interoceptive network, are being sent *from* your body *to* your brain. By training with exercises that focus on using breath, posture and touch, you'll be learning how to use your body to send your brain the messages you want it to receive. We also know that body-up signals influence neuroception, which is a survival brain's job. For simplicity, I've divided these resources according to their desired result:

- **Toolkit 1** (Chapter 9) contains exercises to shift you out of the sympathetic state
- **Toolkit 2** (Chapter 10) contains exercises to shift you out of the dorsal state

I've organised the exercises this way to make it easy for you to find the resources best suited to the state you're in.

Neuroplasticity

As you work through these exercises, you'll be employing one of the most important concepts in any relearning and resetting context: *neuroplasticity*. This is the ability of the neurons in the nervous system – especially the brain – to learn new responses. When we introduce a new experience repeatedly, as you'll be doing by training with these resources, we encourage our neurons to change their structure, functions and connections to reorganise themselves in a new (and ideally, better) way.

The phenomenon of neuroplasticity is most evident throughout our childhood and adolescence as new neurons are growing rapidly, and that's when many new skills become embedded in our nature. The relationships and experiences we have in these early years carve pathways in our nervous system, forming particular responses that become automatic by adulthood. If you grew up with an angry parent who shouted a lot, you might feel scared or heated when others raise their voice around you. That doesn't have to be the way you respond forever, though.

It's become clear relatively recently that neuroplasticity doesn't end when we grow up. It *is* possible to change our brain and nervous system throughout our lives. Thought patterns, expectations and beliefs can cause this. If you've heard of placebo effect, you'll know that believing something to be true and expecting certain results can actually change the body's physiology.

In earlier chapters, we explored the negative, or 'darker' side of bioplasticity, which occurs when our bodily systems get better at trying to keep us safe but overcorrect to the point that we become hypersensitive to danger and develop faulty neuroception. When this happens, we shift into a more extreme state and our vital coping systems – such as our emotional, cognitive, immune, endocrine and autonomic systems – can be switched on for extended periods of time. As we saw in the earlier examples of Sophia (page 48), Tom (page 50) and even my own situation (page 52), this usually happens by accident. It's a by-product of whatever challenging situation or circumstances we find ourselves in.

But just as we have the power to accidentally overcorrect, we also have the power to intentionally redress that balance by taking conscious action. In a fascinating study of a group of London's iconic black cab drivers, brain scans revealed that they had larger than average spatial memory centres (the thinking brain's hippocampi) than the average population. These drivers hadn't been born with enlarged memory centres; the mental demands of their job had caused them to expand.

To acquire the coveted black cab licence, drivers must pass an exam known as 'the knowledge'. This requires them to have an encyclopedic knowledge of more than 25,000 of London's streets, not to mention hundreds of tourist attractions, and how best to navigate to them from any point in the city. To build this knowledge, drivers spend three or four years studying. They memorise maps and routes, but they also spend a lot of time driving around the city and forming that all-important 'experiential' knowledge. In the process, their neurons change and this new information becomes embedded and automatic. This is neuroplasticity in action. The hippocampus is expanding to make room for this new information.

Bioplasticity

The term 'bioplasticity' was coined by physiotherapist Lorimer Moseley to capture the phenomenon of the physical changes that take place when we learn new things. Whether we're learning how to lift weights or taking up a new musical instrument, our neurons change so we can learn the movement patterns required to execute a deadlift or play a certain sequence of notes or chord. But while that's happening, other parts of us are also adapting and learning. Every squat strengthens bones and alters muscular imbalances little by little. Evenings of practising guitar build hand strength and form calluses on fingertips, making it easier for us to manipulate the strings. After enough training, correct form comes naturally, and the placement of our fingers on the strings is automatic because new pathways have formed as we've learned. Knowing how to activate these movements are a result of *neuro*plasticity and we may even see the representation of the hand of the sensory map we introduced on page 142 get larger from this training, but the physical changes happening in tandem with them are a result of *bio*plasticity.

In my career as a physiotherapist, these processes brought me the most rewarding experiences I had with patients. I saw how, with repetition and training, a client in their later years could come back from a debilitating stroke and re-learn vital life skills – walking, talking and using their affected limbs again. As a new mother, plasticity has become a bigger part of my life than I ever anticipated. My daughter had a challenging start in life, and spent several of her first months in and out of hospital. Now that she's home, I take her through daily exercises and marvel at how quickly she's forming the neural pathways needed to remember them. Small movements she couldn't do a few weeks ago get easier and easier until one day, I noticed that they've become second nature. Children's earliest years are considered the 'golden years' when it comes to neuroplasticity because they are growing and 'pruning' neurons – their brains are highly adaptable.

Although some central nervous system injuries like stroke, traumatic brain injury, and spinal cord injury cause long-term disability, the way the human brain and body is able to work together to reorganise and transform itself in these ways is one of our greatest superpowers. And in the same way our muscles and bones can become stronger through training, we can also train our nervous system to make it more flexible, adaptable and resilient. Life circumstances may have wired you to respond in certain ways, but that doesn't mean you're stuck with that wiring. Through bioplasticity, you can recalibrate a dysregulated and overprotective nervous system and relearn how to respond to life in a more balanced and regulated way.

This nervous system training isn't complicated, either. The exercises I'm going to be sharing with you are straightforward, accessible and quick. And when performed regularly, they gently nudge the nervous system towards regulation so it learns to respond to what's actually happening in the present moment rather than defaulting to a position of excess protection, which becomes our response during periods of chronic or traumatic stress.

True learning is not passive, it comes from *doing*. That's why it's not enough for London's cab drivers to memorise a map, they've got to drive the streets until the landmarks and routes become hardwired. If you want to learn to speak a new language, reading vocabulary books isn't enough. You need to practise speaking those new words again and again so your tongue can learn how to move in order to elicit the correct sound.

Experiential learning will be taking place every time you

practise the exercises in the coming chapters. They are the best route to resetting your nervous system, and the only way to widen your window of tolerance, strengthen that vagal tone, and retrain your brain.

Four ingredients for a successful nervous system reset

The principles of plasticity tell us that if we can create a new compelling, embodied experience, we can teach our brain–body system that it can, in fact, cope under stress. Mastering a skill, whether it's speaking a new language or learning to ski, requires training with four key elements in mind, and resetting the nervous system is no different. While practising the tools of self-regulation, be aware of these four elements: specificity, repetition, intensity and time. If you realise that one or more of them is missing from the particular practice you're engaged in, ask yourself how you can tweak things to include them.

1. Specificity

The methods we use to regulate the connection between the brain and body should be tailored to the current state of our nervous system. In simpler terms, the approach to healing and transformation needs to match the specific requirements of our nervous system at any given time. In the context of physical fitness, setting very specific goals is usually the first step before training starts. Rather than saying you want to build strength, you might decide that you want lower trapezius muscles so your shoulder posture improves. If that's the case, the exercises you practise will be the ones that target those specific muscles. Similarly, if you're stuck in a cold state, your goal might be to focus on practising the specific exercises and tools that will pull you out of that cold state and into your window of tolerance.

When I found myself stuck in an oscillating state between hot and cold, the interoception skills I'd started developing made it possible for me to identify that I was spending most of my time in the dorsal vagal state. So I started there, and zeroed in on the tools I needed to pull me out of that specific state. I found that using movement-based tools, such as walking or going to the park, whenever I found I was unable to motivate myself, had the power to snap me out of that dorsal vagal state by raising my heart rate and blood pressure and giving me a much-needed injection of energy. The more I practised that tool, the easier it became to pull myself out of that colder state before I could get stuck too far in it. This may not have worked when I was in the sympathetic nervous system state as it wasn't specific to where my nervous system was.

Specificity doesn't just refer to the tool, however; it also relates to our ability to get more granular about the things we're feeling and thinking. With better interoceptive skills and autonomic awareness comes the ability to go beyond vague descriptions and notice more subtle sensations, feelings and patterns. Instead of feeling 'unwell', you might notice that your stomach is gurgling and your face feels flushed. The more specifically you can pinpoint your bodily signals, the more likely you are to find the right tool to regulate them.

2. Repetition

Building new skills and carving new pathways requires repetition, ideally daily repetition. The soccer player who spends an hour each day kicking balls at a goal is more likely to create deep muscle memory, which in turn makes them more likely to score under pressure on game day than their teammate who practises a few times a week. Similarly, establishing a daily practice where you tune in to your body by following a calming breathing routine makes it much more likely that you'll slip into that routine in moments where you most need to feel calm. It helps us in the heat of the moment if we have 'rehearsed' before the going gets tough.

3. Intensity

Stretching intensity

While repetition is essential to creating new pathways, anything we do regularly will eventually become routine. In order to grow, we must 'load' our system by performing the same exercise in more challenging ways. A runner looking to improve their endurance might choose to load their system by running up hills rather than at their track. To increase vagal tone and strength, you can load your nervous system by using the tools you learn in the moment (i.e. when you're feeling flustered, angry, sad or collapsed) as well as during your regular practice (i.e. when you're in a regulated state). This ups the intensity of the exercises and takes you into your 'stretch zone'. Keep in mind, though, your stretch zone is at the *edge* of your window of tolerance, not outside it.

Emotional intensity

How much you get out of your training and the amount of transformation that occurs in your brain–body system will depend on what that training means to you – your *why*, if you will. This is because emotions can modulate the intensity of the training as well as the memory consolidation. Simply put, you're more likely to remember things if they relate to something that's important to you, especially if your nervous system is already overwhelmed. A child who loves the outdoors might learn how to pitch a tent and build a campfire in one day, yet take weeks to master a simple piano scale because they have no deep desire to learn an instrument.

A stroke patient who loses strength in one arm might be motivated to restore strength so they can grip utensils and cook with their family again. Their desire to get back to doing an activity they love with people who are important to them might well make the patient more willing to stretch themselves physically in rehabilitation sessions. In this scenario, emotional intensity is likely to fuel their determination and help their brain and body consolidate the muscle memory required for certain movements faster than patients who aren't emotionally motivated.

As I mentioned at the start of the book, your intentions and goals – your *why?* – play a pivotal role in your nervous system reset. To achieve real and lasting change, your goal must be something that is important to you.

4. Time

We live in a world of instant gratification, but in the same way that building muscle, losing weight or becoming good at a sport takes time, we must also accept and remind ourselves that plasticity is a long game rather than a single event we can quickly tick off our to-do list. Success depends on consistency, patience and time.

Towards healthy interoception

In Chapter 7 we'll be building your interoception 'muscles' so you can get better at noticing when you're becoming angry, anxious, collapsed or shut down. This awareness gives you an opportunity to manage your emotions by taking action that prevents you from entering into dysregulation in the first place.

Healthy interoception allows us to make decisions based on logic and emotions.

Without healthy interoception, we'd be stuck having to carefully think through every possible response and outcome to every situation. Basing decisions on logic alone is extremely tiring, and contributes to rumination, overload, shutdown, meltdowns, anxiety and depression. There are so many benefits to building strong interoceptive skills. With better interoception you'll have access to:

- balanced input as to what's happening in the present moment
- information you can use to guide you in your present-day life
- strong inner knowing, which fosters greater self-confidence
- greater trust in your abilities, including when you're outside your comfort zone
- a more even way of operating
- the understanding that your responsibility isn't to be perfect, but rather to work to the best of your ability
- the power of saying no in order to take care of your own needs

- clarity about the reality of any given situation and what your intentions are
- awareness of where you are in relation to your limits
- agency and control.

Understanding theory and cognitive learning is essential, but being *in* our body is equally essential, and perhaps more so. The science suggests that too much interoceptive awareness when we're dysregulated can exacerbate anxiety and depression. So instead:

The goal is to get to a state where we can practise interoception and tune in, then switch fluidly to exteroception so we can add more context to those sensations and use our body to respond or regulate.

The better we become at returning to our window of tolerance, the better our body will be at mitigating some of the wear and tear caused by life's stresses. Our natural balance will be restored, and our systems will function more optimally.

7

Start where you are: Mapping your nervous system states

So much information about the nervous system states and the way we fluctuate between them is abstract and academic. And while knowledge is great, we've already established that it's not enough to create meaningful change. For that, we need to apply what we *know* to our daily reality. The only way to reset our nervous system, widen our window of tolerance and come home to our centre is through experiential learning. In other words, we have to *feel* what it's like to be within each state, and also what it feels like to come home to our set point. This is what will help us establish a baseline and build autonomic awareness of our internal nervous system functions. We call this process 'mapping the states'.

The first step in this process involves using interoceptive skills to interpret what's going on inside you and which state you're in. I'm sure you know how good it feels when someone understands how you feel and where you're coming from. Well, you can offer that same feeling of comfort and belonging to yourself by tuning in to what's going on inside of you.

Like a fingerprint, your nervous system is completely unique, so before you attempt to reset it, you have to get to know it. As you become more skilled at listening to this self-communicating system, you'll become better at accurately interpreting the messages it's sending. This is powerful, because it means you'll become better at distinguishing between *real* threats and *perceived* threats.

When tuning in is hard

Our ability to override our gut instincts or tune out bodily signals for the sake of survival is an incredible adaptation. But when we override these signals for an extended period – to cope with an ongoing crisis, for example – we can dull our interoceptive abilities, making it harder for us to notice those signals in the future.

If you've been dissociated from your body for quite some time, it can take time to re-learn how to tune in to yourself again, and we want to do this in a trauma-informed way. Start small and practise tuning in only when you're within your window of tolerance. Using exteroceptive resources such as tapping or touch may also be helpful, as the sensory information from our skin is less overwhelming than that coming from our organs, which may flood us and our survival brain with emotions. We can also switch to noticing sensations in areas of the body that feel pleasant or neutral, such as the hands and feet.

Neurodivergent individuals can experience bodily signals as sensations that are either 'too loud' or 'too quiet'. As a result, it can be challenging for them to interpret their signals. If this is you, you can use touch and movement to help you connect with your signals.

For example, you might find it easy to connect with the beats of your heart after walking uphill. The exercises in this chapter are a good place to start. You may also lean into co-regulation or seek feedback from a healthcare professional to help you get started.

Map your just-right state

Let's start by mapping your window of tolerance – that just-right state. Exploring how you feel when you're most at ease and at your set point will give you a baseline from which to view the other two states. If you've never mapped or assessed your nervous system like this before, don't put too much pressure on yourself. Building autonomic awareness is important, but it's not a process you should rush. You can revisit the following exercises over and over as you hone your interoceptive skills and get better at recognising and interpreting the messages your body is sending.

Practising interoception helps us cultivate agency and notice when we've moved beyond our physiological capabilities and limits. When we ignore those signals and push through regardless, we override our neurobiological limits and allostasis stops working properly because we don't return to our baseline, and this is the hallmark of dysregulation.

If you notice an increase in heart rate or a worsening of your anxiety while mapping a particular state, that doesn't mean you're doing the exercise wrong or that there's something wrong with you. People with a history of trauma can sometimes find that sitting in stillness feels unsafe. On paper, that might seem strange, but if we look at this response from a biological point of view, it makes a lot of sense. After all, if stillness is how your body tells your brain that you're vulnerable, your brain is bound to reply by yelling, 'We need to escape!' If you're sitting still to map your state, forcing yourself to stay that way isn't going to help you get to know this state, it's only going to create more panic and dissociation. Take those signals as a cue to find an approach that suits you better. You may find it helpful to work with a trauma-informed health professional if getting started with interoception proves too challenging. This could include a physiotherapist, osteopath, chiropractor or massage therapist who can help you connect to your body with postural corrections or manual therapy, or it could be a psychologist or psychotherapist. Alternatively, you could start by just noticing the postures that your body moves into (aka proprioceptive information).

Exercise: Find your window of tolerance

Take out your notebook or journal and work through the following nine steps. Alternatively, use my worksheet at www.jessicamaguire.com/mapping.

1. Create an outline for the three states

On a blank piece of paper, draw three wide rows – the middle row should be the widest. This middle row represents your window of tolerance, so label this section 'Just right'. The upper row should be labelled 'Too hot' and the bottom row 'Too cold'. As you work through the exercises on the following pages, write down everything you feel and notice in each state. Any changes in bodily sensations, emotions, posture, gestures, movements and thoughts are worth noting. If internal stories come up while you're in a certain state, write those down too. Each piece of information forms part of your unique nervous system roadmap.

2. Actively embody your just-right state

Since you're currently reading (or listening to an audiobook) and likely sitting still, you're hopefully already within your window of tolerance and feeling calm, relaxed and at ease. If not, let's try to get into that state now. First, find a comfortable position – lie down or sit in a way you find relaxing. Next, visualise a time when you felt a strong sense of safety, trust and connection – to yourself, to others or to the environment around you. Picture this scenario in as much detail as possible for a couple of minutes to give your body time to settle into this environment. If nothing comes to mind, use one of these prompts to recall an image in detail:

- a walk with a friend or loved one
- a conversation in which you really felt seen and heard
- a hike through the forest, a day at the beach, floating in a lake, or a visit to place where you felt a deep sense of connection
- completing a project that made you feel connected to your sense of self.

3. Reflect on your physical sensations

Now, allow your focus to shift from imagining that scenario, to your body. Start at one end of your body and take a mental inventory of how your body responds to being in this just-right state. Consider these questions:

- Are your breaths full and easy?
- Is your heartbeat slow or fast?
- What is your jaw doing?

- How does your tongue feel in your mouth?
- Is your belly soft?

4. Reflect on your emotions

Give yourself time to identify anything you're experiencing, then write that down in the widest row of your piece of paper. Some people describe feeling:

- connected
- warm
- spacious
- expansive
- secure
- safe
- calm.

5. Gauge your energy

Notice if your body's energy feels more mobilised or immobilised. This could be subtle:

- nervousness
- mild irritation
- a 'daydream' fog
- sleepiness.

Or it could be compelling:

- anxious
- agitated
- hypervigilant
- collapsed
- exhausted
- apathetic.

6. Examine your posture

- Is your posture open or closed? If your arms are folded and your knees are touching or thigh muscles are tense, see you if you can let your hands relax into your lap. Then, let your body be supported by the chair your sitting in.
- Are your shoulders soft or tense? If you notice tension, can you lift your shoulders slowly up then, even slower, let them lower, focusing on the kinaesthetic information of that slow softening. You might visualise ice melting into water.
- Is your spine bracing or slumped? If you notice bracing, let yourself rotate side to side before relaxing your spine against the chair. If you're slumped, see if you can move into a posture where you're both alert and relaxed. Rolling up a small towel and placing it under the 'sitting bone' at the back of the pelvis will help the spine to line up. The position of your shoulders and spine is especially important for the breath, which also impacts the nervous system.

7. Go deeper

Exaggerate any of the subtle bodily changes you just noticed so you can *feel* what it's like to shift into your just-right state even further. If you noticed that your jaw softened, loosen it more. If your shoulders are down, can you relax them a touch more? If you felt a sense of arriving in your body when you adjusted your spine, continue to notice this. All of these 'body-up' messages are signalling to the survival brain that things are safe and well, this will help you continue to shift towards regulation.

8. Observe your thoughts

You may find it helpful to reimagine yourself in the situation or scenario where you felt a sense of safety and connection. As you go deeper into this, spend a minute or two observing your thoughts and writing them down. Answer the following questions if you're not sure where to start.

- Are your thoughts manageable and not overwhelming?
- Are they slowing down?
- Are they becoming more expansive and optimistic?
- Have any worries or stories around shame started to dissipate?
- If you felt foggy and dissociated from the present moment are your thoughts now becoming clearer?

9. Drop a pin in this location

Now that you're within your window of tolerance and operating from a calm, sociable place, write down on a separate page how you're feeling emotionally and physically. Take note of your breathing and heart rate, and articulate as best as you can how being calm and centred feels for you. Label this description 'Centring resource', and add to it as you gather more information in the future.

Throughout the day, try to notice the sensations you feel when you're inside this window, and work on your capacity to notice and name your various sensations with specificity. If you notice a warm feeling when you share a smile with your barista or say hi to your neighbour, note that down. If chatting to someone in your office elicits a sense of connection or belonging, make a note of that and use that information to help inch you back to your set point next time you feel lonely.

Taking these tiny steps towards regulation can have lasting positive effects on your nervous system. The more skilled you become at noticing and then identifying how your body functions in your just-right state, the easier it will be to find your way back to it when you spend too long in the hot or cold state.

From interoception to exteroception: The key to nervous system training

It bears repeating that one of the primary goals of nervous system training is to learn to shift dynamically between interoception and exteroception when we choose to. An example of this could be during a time of conflict with another person who's dysregulated. We notice what's going on with the other person, and then reconnect to our internal experience – this can help us stay centred. If things escalate and we feel like we're about to move into rage or flip our lid, we might leave the room and focus on what we notice with our outer-facing senses: what we see, hear, smell or the points of our body making contact with a chair or the environment. Mapping your nervous system helps you to recognise early on what your emotional states are so you can pro-actively manage them. Without this skill we may not notice the irritation turning into anger, until we say or do something that we don't mean.

Let's try that again now, this time in a hotter, more activated state.

 Map your too hot state

Now that you've mapped your set point, let's explore more turbulent territory. Our bodily systems are inextricably linked, so feeling physical responses when moving into your too hot sympathetic state is perfectly normal.

Exercise: Find your too hot state

1. Actively embody your too hot state

Assuming you're not already in this too hot state, let's try to embody that now. Bring to mind a time when you noticed that this hotter side of you had been activated. Start with something that made you feel anxious but not overwhelmed. It won't serve you here to pick something traumatic – we're just looking to start with something that we can work with to get to know this state. Perhaps you recently found yourself defending a person or topic you feel passionate about, or maybe you experienced a stressful situation that made you feel angry or argumentative.

Once you've got something in mind, spend a few minutes recalling this memory in as much detail as possible so you can put yourself back in that moment. If nothing comes to mind, think of any upcoming events or situations. Whatever you choose, put yourself in that scenario and embody the feelings it brings as much as possible.

2. Reflect on your physical sensations

Scan your body to find out how it's responding to this perceived stress. Write anything you notice in the top row of map you drew up earlier, above the notes you made for your just-right state. Use the following questions as prompts and write down anything you're noticing:

- Is your jaw clenched?
- Is your brow furrowed?
- Are you squeezing your eyes shut?
- Has your heart rate increased?
- Do you notice heat or a constriction in your chest?

- Do you feel a clenching in your torso?
- How is your breath?
- Is there tightness in your hips and legs?
- Are you experiencing a sense of urgency that's making it hard to sit still?

3. Reflect on your emotions

Now, spend a few moments noticing the emotions arising within you. Dig into whatever it is you're feeling and get as specific as possible when naming your emotion(s). Write your observations in the top row of your piece of paper. Which of these emotions are most prevalent now that you've entered this state?

- Irritation.
- Nervousness.
- Agitation.
- Anxiousness.
- Fear.
- Anger.
- Rage.
- Spite.
- Rebelliousness.
- Malice.

It's common to try to push strong emotions like these away, but see if you can allow them to just be. The point here isn't to make you more uncomfortable, it's to make you more resilient. Developing our ability to not turn away from unpleasant stimuli helps us improve our survival brain's functioning during stress arousal and intense emotions. Noticing these signals early on is how you then can take steps to change things in your life.

Remember, we also want to do this in a trauma-informed way. When you need to stop, it's wise to listen to your body.

4. Gauge your energy

In the sympathetic nervous system state our energy is mobilised. Ask yourself if any of these describe the activation in your nervous system:

- tightly wound up
- hyperactive
- overstimulated
- agitated
- unable to sit still
- fidgety.

5. Examine your posture

Sometimes when fight or flight takes over we're not aware of the reflexive changes our body makes. Notice how you are holding yourself and consider these questions:

- Are you tense?
- Are you pacing around the room or do you feel like it?
- Does your neck feel stiff?
- Are your shoulders lifted?
- Do you notice bracing in your rib cage?
- Are your hands balled into fists?
- Is your stomach constricted?

6. Go deeper

Now I want you to lean in to and exaggerate some of the physical reactions you've noticed. Give in to what your body is urging you to do and whatever position or posture you're already holding. Go further. Exaggerate the change in posture so you can strengthen your brain–body connection: clench your jaw harder, tense your shoulders, make fists with your hands, stand up or hug yourself tighter.

Close your eyes or soften your gaze and look down. As you do, focus your mind on the stressful situation you're imagining and consider the following questions:

- Do you have an urge to fight or express anger?
- Do you want to run away or towards something?
- What is it that your body is wanting to do to express what's happening?

Some physical reactions will be more obvious than others, but even subtle changes are worth writing down. As you bring your attention to these sensations, I invite you to put your hand on the area where they're occurring. The sensation of touch can help increase interoceptive awareness of sensations by drawing our attention to that area even more.

7. Observe your thoughts

Still picturing this stressful scenario, reflect on the details.

- Who are you with?
- What are you doing?

Pause on the exact moment you find most challenging. You might even name what that is aloud or whisper it to yourself.

- 'What am I believing?'
- 'What stories am I telling about myself? Do I believe them?'
- 'When I'm believing this thought or narrative, what changes do I notice in my body?'

8. Drop a pin in this location

Once you finish examining your thoughts, grab your notebook or journal and on a fresh page near your centring resource list write a few sentences articulating what being in this too hot state feels like for you. Add to this paragraph and to your map when new situations carry you into this state. The more detail you can add to your map, the better. After completing this mapping exercise you may find it useful to go for a fast walk to discharge some of the mobilising energy that you brought into your nervous system with this activity. Something that gets your heart rate up for 10 minutes can be enough – your neuroendocrine system hormones have just encouraged the release of glucose for energy. It can be helpful to burn some of it off so you return to regulation. As we'll soon discover, movement is one of the most effective body-up regulating resources.

Map your too cold state

Now, it's time to map your too cold dorsal vagal state. You may discover this is a frequent state for you, so it's important to know what it feels like.

Exercise: Find your too cold state

1. Actively embody your too cold state

In order to experience your too cold state, recall a time, perhaps recently, when you felt helpless and hopeless. It could be a time that brought up some shame and a feeling of being alone and disconnected from others. Whether this experience was related to work, family or something else entirely, I invite you to sink into this moment and fully immerse yourself in that memory. Again, I don't want you to pick anything traumatic such as a death or an injury. You're just looking for an experience that was mildly painful so you can drop yourself into this state and understand it.

If you need some help thinking of a scenario, here are examples of experiences that might cause us to move into the dorsal vagal state:

- A friend didn't return your call.
- You weren't invited to a social outing.
- You were reprimanded at work.
- You had a fight with your partner that left you feeling alone.
- The bank declined a loan you desperately needed.

Once you've chosen your memory, picture it playing again like a movie in your mind. Close your eyes, visualise the experience in detail, and pause for a moment.

2. Reflect on your physical sensations

Once you've assessed the physical sensations in your body, notice what urges it has.

- Does your body want you to collapse through the spine?
- Do you want to drop your head?
- Do you want to lie down?

3. Reflect on your emotions

Once in the moment, consider the emotions the sensations you're experiencing are giving rise to. Do your best to notice them, and try to be as specific as possible. You might feel:

- numb
- blue
- lonely
- shame
- disconnected
- hollow
- hopeless.

4. Gauge your energy

In the sympathetic nervous system state our energy is immobilised. This could be just the dorsal vagal 'collapse' energy, or it might be freeze – predominantly a dorsal vagal state, but there could also be sympathetic activation. Ask yourself if any of these describe the activation in your nervous system:

- collapsed
- exhausted
- stuck
- frozen
- in cement.

5. Observe your posture

- How are you holding yourself?
- Are you slumped in a chair or lying down?
- Do you feel heavy and that you can't hold yourself up?
- Do your shoulders sag?

6. Go deeper into this state

Lean in to whatever position you're holding and exaggerate some of the physical reactions you've noticed. Give in to what your body is urging you to do and exaggerate the change in posture so you can strengthen your brain–body connection. Let your head drop, your spine collapse, your face go blank. If you're sitting down, you might even let yourself lie down on a couch or bed.

Close your eyes or soften your gaze and look down. As you do, focus even more on the stressful situation in your mind and consider the following questions:

- Do you have an urge to move into helplessness or give up?
- Do you notice any feelings of shame?

7. Observe your thoughts

Finally, consider the thoughts and stories that are running through your mind as you're in this state. Do the stories and thoughts you're telling about yourself revolve around:

- hopelessness and apathy
- failure and lack of belonging
- loneliness and isolation
- shame?

You might even name what that is aloud or whisper it to yourself.

- 'What am I believing?'
- 'What stories am I telling about myself? Do I believe them?'
- 'When I'm believing this thought or narrative, what changes do I notice in my body?'

8. Drop a pin in this location

Now that you've considered your thoughts and feelings, it's time to map this state. While in this state:

- How did your body respond?
- How did your posture shift?
- What were your thoughts and stories like?

Take as long as you need and write everything down, no matter how subtle or insignificant you think the sensation or thought might be. Even things like a sense of disconnection from your surroundings or the vague feeling that you might float away are crucial to note, because survival states take us out of the present moment.

Again, movement can be useful after mapping this state but you may choose gentle rocking, rhythmical movement to fully up-regulate yourself to the just-right state. You could try lying on your back and gently rocking your knees side to side. Then move into standing and let your weight shift from one foot to the other rocking slowly.

Map your secondary states

Remember, we're not just dealing with the three primary states, we also spend a great deal of our lives between states, in what we call a secondary or blended state (see pages 55–57). Like those primary states, blended states are also highly individual, so getting to know how you feel when in each of them is equally important. As you work through each mapping exercise below, make notes in your notebook or diary of any feelings or physical sensations these secondary states arouse.

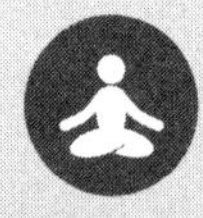

Exercise: Map your play state 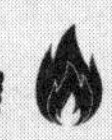

When we're in this state, we may feel secure and happy. We could also feel excited, motivated, ready for action or in our flow state. We're within our window of tolerance, but at the higher edge of it – with access to the energy of the hotter state.

To actively embody your play state, think of a time when you felt mobilised and full of positive energy? Bring this memory to mind and see if you can feel its influence on your brain–body system.

- What bodily signals do you notice?
- What emotions do those sensations give rise to?
- Do you notice any changes to your thoughts, focus or clarity?

Make a note of your answers in your notebook or journal so that you can recognise your play state next time you encounter it.

The importance of vagal tone

If we don't have good vagal tone, we may lose our ability to get into our play state and feel excited while also staying within our window of tolerance. When this is the case, the spark of excitement that should shift us into the play state is more likely to carry us into fear of the hot state. Instead of feeling playful and energetic, we're likely to end up feeling anxious or overwhelmed.

To get ourselves into a play state, we can practise accessing mobilising energy while in a stretch zone and inside our window of tolerance. Write a list of activities you find fun and energising, then engage in them when you're in your window of tolerance. Get involved enough that you can get carried away by the activity while still feeling safe. This could be playing a game of basketball or tennis with friends, running in the park with your dog, or playing a few games of Jenga with a child.

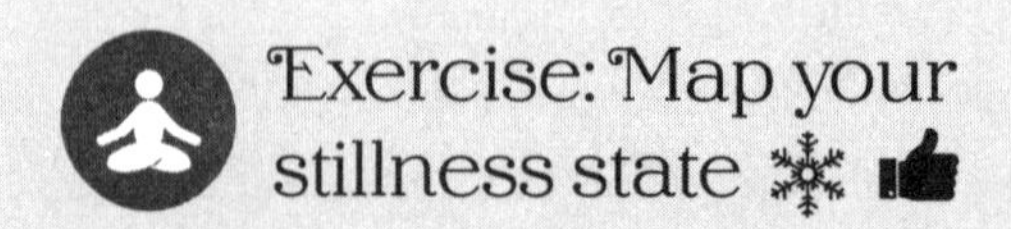

Exercise: Map your stillness state

To actively embody your stillness state, think of a time when you felt the immobilising energy of that too cold state but also a sense of safety and connection. It could be a time when you were deeply relaxed, like at the end of a massage or yoga class, or when you were almost asleep or breastfeeding. It could even be as you lay close with someone. Bring this memory from your stillness state to mind and see if you can feel its influence on your brain–body system.

- What bodily signals do you notice?
- What emotions do those sensations give rise to?
- Do you notice any changes to your thoughts, focus or clarity?

Given how calm and relaxing the stillness state is, you might assume it's one that everyone would welcome, but as we saw earlier, that isn't always the case. Someone with a history of trauma may find that forcing themselves to remain still and power through whatever supposedly calming activity they're doing can actually lead them to experience more panic and dissociation. There's no perfect practice or one silver-bullet exercise that works for everyone. Only by mapping the topography of your own inner landscape can you determine which tools will work best for you and when.

Your roadmap to nervous system regulation

Congratulations! You now have a fairly detailed roadmap of your unique nervous system as it exists today. Having everything down will help you to recognise the landmarks in each state and orient yourself more easily as you move between them. Intentionally experiencing every state the way you've just done is how you begin to truly feel the boundaries of your own window of tolerance, and sense when you're about to step outside them. Having this baseline will help you to keep your window of tolerance wide and allow you to maintain equilibrium in the face of stressful or traumatic events.

Embodying each one of your states helps you learn what's happening in your nervous system. It opens your awareness to the subtle changes that occur when you shift between states in an embodied rather than a cognitive way. This lifelong skill, which you can continue to hone, is the key to regaining your agency and reshaping your responses to stressful situations as they occur.

If you weren't able to embody the states, look for clues

If you tried to map your states but you can't embody them all quite yet, all is not lost. You'll be able to do this with time and practise, and in the meantime you can find clues to your dominant state (i.e. the one you spend the most time in) in your health, behaviour and thought patterns. If you suspect that you're dysregulated, this diagram might help you figure out if you're in that too hot or too cold zone.

Too hot!

'I'm going to fail.' hyper vigilance starting arguments

'Things will fall apart.' digestive problems insomnia

Stretch zone

Just right

'The world is a safe place.' rest and recovery

'I'm connected and safe.' attaching and connecting with others growth and restoration

Stretch zone

Too cold!

'It never works out for me.' isolating self forgetfulness

'There's no use trying, I give up.' apathy extreme fatigue immune issues

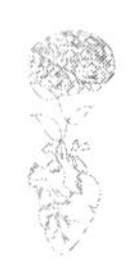

Now that you have your map, you can gauge which tools you'll need to bring yourself back into your window of tolerance. But first, let's take a look at how you might go about choosing those tools.

8

Choosing the right tools for the right job

Nervous system regulation becomes possible when we listen to, and then honour, our own needs. But if we don't understand how our nervous system functions or know how to find out what it needs, we're likely to keep using the wrong tools to shift our state. As we've already seen, artificial regulators such as alcohol, social media, video games, drugs or sex might make us feel a little better in the short term, but they don't work in the long run. When we're grabbing onto the wrong tools, they can take us further away from our set point and even increase the dysregulation we're trying to escape.

When we're dysregulated, it's human nature to look for ways to feel better. This is why we all develop coping strategies of one sort or another. But when these strategies do us more harm than good, we suffer negative consequences on so many fronts – from our gut microbiota to our mental health, heart health and lifestyle. This makes us feel worse, and the cycle continues.

Exercise: Break down your emotion regulators

If you're aware that you're using artificial regulators to cope with your life, this is a good time to become curious as to why. Use the worksheet below (or download a version at www.jessicamaguire.com/regulators) to help you work out when you reach for those crutches, how they help you in the moment and what needs might be driving your go-to coping mechanisms.

1. Identify a habit you use to artificially regulate your nervous system

This could, for example, be social media scrolling. Answer the following questions:

- Which nervous system state are you in?
- Can you notice the bodily signals, emotions, thoughts and urges of that state?
- How long or how often are you using this as a coping mechanism? Perhaps it's three, four or five hours a day.
- What triggers lead you to use this coping mechanism? Do certain people, environments, situations or emotions that cause you, say, to reach for your phone? You might notice, for example, that this happens at night time when you feel alone.

2. Examine the short-term benefits this artificial regulator provides

Answer the following questions to guide you through:

- Does it relieve or soothe your nervous system?
- Does it fill an emptiness?

For example, using social media on your phone might deliver

a few benefits, such as helping you numb out from everything you need to do (artificially downregulating). If you're lonely, it might give you a connection to other people or a sense of belonging. Or it might be a distraction or bring some kind of excitement if you feel helpless or hopeless about your current work situation (artificially upregulating).

3. Identify your unmet need

This is where you can look below the surface and see what's going on in the bulk of the iceberg (see page 12). Your answers to this question will most likely link to whichever state you're in.

As you work through each of your top coping mechanisms, consider if there are other, more positive, actions you could take to meet your nervous system's true needs. For example, if you know that you use social media because it gives you a sense of connection (and it *can* sometimes bring a feeling of belonging), this suggests that you could be in that colder dorsal vagal state, and feeling lonely and disconnected. Could phoning a friend soothe that loneliness? Would listening to an interesting podcast and going to the park where there are other people in your community make you feel more connected than mindlessly scrolling? Do you need to schedule a walk with your friends?

Perhaps social media gives you a jolt of excitement that counters feelings of boredom and emptiness. This, too, suggests that you might be in a colder state and would benefit from some other form of upregulating. A healthier way of meeting your need for fulfillment and excitement might be swapping your phone for the pottery wheel in your garage so you can finally launch that side hustle you've been fantasising about. Or it could be using some gentle movement.

Alternatively, you might like using social media because it distracts you from the impossibly high standards you've set for yourself and helps you escape from your reality. A better way to shift yourself out of that hotter sympathetic nervous system state and regulate the tension your perfectionism is creating might involve delegating work to your teammates, helping your clients to have more realistic expectations, or talking to your boss about your demanding schedule.

To make a note of your discoveries with this exercise, you might draw up a table like the one below. Your unmet needs will tell you what your nervous system truly needs, and what part of your reality your artificial coping mechanism is preventing you from seeing.

Habit	**What short-term benefits does it provide**	**What's my unmet need?**	**Action**
Social media scrolling (3 hours on Saturdays)	1. I can numb out from everything I need to do.	The expectations I've set for myself at work are too high.	Review my deadlines, delegate, ask for help, lower my expectations.
	2. Connection to others, a sense of belonging.	Since I started working from home, I've been feeling lonely and isolated.	Phone an old friend for a catch-up.
	3. Excitement and distraction.	I'm unfulfilled in my work.	Research writing/ pottery/ business courses.

Why finding the right tool is so important

The interesting thing about gathering resources to help you with your nervous system reset is that even tools that *do* work for regulation can trip you up if you use them in the wrong context. Take mindfulness, for example. It's a brilliant practice that's been scientifically proven to improve wellness on several fronts. But that doesn't mean it's the best tool for everyone in all moments. If, for example, you're stuck in a dorsal vagal state and experiencing an impending sense of doom, it may lead you to dissociate from your body further if you focus on those sensations and force yourself to be still. Stillness and being mindful of the impending sense of doom you feel can be interpreted by your survival brain as a threat, and may increase your stress levels even more. Or, if you're in the hot sympathetic nervous system state and you start paying attention to feeling that you can't breathe when your panicked or like your heart is going to explode out of your chest, this may amplify dysregulation. If you force yourself to sit still and focus when your system wants to mobilise and move, this may not be what serves you best. You might even get frustrated and blame yourself, and think things like, *How come mindfulness works so well for that woman on Instagram but not me? I must be doing something wrong.*

Too often we reach for the wrong tool, either because we don't understand the state it's designed for, or because we haven't tuned in to what's actually happening inside our body. If we don't like the way we're feeling, we're impatient and want results, so we grab the first shiny tool we see.

This is why the first step in your nervous system reset will be tracking your nervous system regularly. Being able to identify what temperature your thermostat is set to at any given moment is *the* best way I know to engage your interoceptive network and build this skill. As you do so, you'll also be accumulating the resources to help you re-regulate your nervous system. By tuning in to yourself regularly, you'll get better at choosing the right tools for your needs.

After that, the next step will be learning which tools to use in which state. There are lots of them, and they're simple to master and easy to use. As I've already mentioned, the nervous system loves choice, and there's plenty of that coming up.

When it comes to plasticity, the fewer tools the better

Since there are many, many ways of working with the vagus nerve, you may be surprised to read that we'll only be focusing on 20 of them, but I assure you, there are several good reasons for this. For one thing, by practising a selected number of tools over and over, you'll be honouring the principles of plasticity, which require a great deal of repetition for change to occur.

The likelihood of you practising a multitude of exercises (more than what we're covering) often enough to create new pathways is pretty slim. With fewer tools, you'll have time to learn how to use each one properly, understand its function, and repeat whichever ones work best for you frequently enough that they become instinctive. This becomes especially important during moments of stress.

When you're in an activated state, a tool you've used again and again will spring to mind straight away and be easier to access than exercises you only vaguely know how to do. That's not to say you can't master all the tools in this book and then add more to your toolkits in the future (in fact, you can check out more on my webpage for this book, www.jessicamaguire.com/reset). To start, though, just trust me that less is more.

Unlike external resources from friends, peers or community members, the tools in the following chapters are internal ones that you can use anytime and anywhere to manage and regulate your nervous system. These tools are part of the way you can train your brain–body system and transform your health by resetting your nervous system.

If we want to achieve masterful regulation and resilience, we need resources that will give us tangible, noticeable results. As you know, your nervous system is inextricably linked to your physical sensations and symptoms. So when dysregulation pulls you outside of your natural set point, tools that can help you alter those sensations and send bodily signals to calm your system are essential for bringing you back inside your window of tolerance.

Bioplasticity tools

Many of the tools we use to come back inside our window of tolerance involve using our body in ways that elicit certain responses from the brain–body system. The term *bioplasticity tools* encompasses the way they integrate the body and brain as one interconnected system to create lasting change. As we previously discussed, neuroplasticity only refers to neurons changing – and so much more transforms when we recalibrate our set point as we've discovered by looking at the immune, endocrine, digestive and cardiovascular systems, just to name a few. It's also more than just body-only tools, without the brain-down aspect we miss the big picture of a nervous system reset and how it transforms the implicit memory system. As we've also discovered from the interoceptive network, our thoughts and beliefs impact how we experience emotions and physical pain.

These resources are designed to send body-up signals of safety to the brain, and train both the body *and* brain to respond to situations accurately. In addition to the interoceptive training you'll be doing whenever you tune in to your bodily signals, you'll be learning exercises that fall under the following four categories:

1. Breathing
2. Posture
3. Containment (tapping or touch)
4. Co-regulation.

As you work through these experiential learning exercises, remember there's no one-size-fits-all approach. Far from it. The exercise that snaps your friend out of a bad mood without fail may not have the same effect on you. Different seasons of your life will shift you into different states. If you're going through a divorce, for example, you may spend long periods of time grieving and feeling shut down and abandoned, in that dorsal vagal state. Alternatively, you may feel highly anxious or angry. You may even oscillate between the two. In this case, something that calmed your nerves at your first job out of school may not do the trick. If you try an exercise and it doesn't do much for you today, don't discount it completely. Tuck it away in your back pocket and revisit it from time to time – especially if your go-to strategies stop working. Years, even decades from now, that tool might become the one thing that *does* work for you.

When we shift outside our window of tolerance, many of us respond in physically unique ways and use resources without realising that's what we're doing. When worried, you might rub your hands along the tops of your thighs or have the sudden urge to go for a jog. You might have a habit of cracking your knuckles or playing with the chain around your neck when nervous. These physical behaviours are your unique way of trying to calm your nervous system.

As we walk through these exercises and assess our responses to them, you'll likely discover a few key bioplasticity resources that will become part of your own nervous system toolbox. The more you use the tools in your toolbox, the more natural they'll become. And as they become habitual, you'll find yourself becoming more resilient and centred.

1. Breathing to support the nervous system

Please note, if you have a respiratory condition, cardiovascular disease (CVD) or a heart condition, please seek professional medical advice regarding the suitability of using breathing tools to support your nervous system reset.

Consciously changing our breathing alters the body-up communication being sent from the respiratory system and influences the brain regions that regulate emotion, thoughts and even behaviour. Some research indicates that it may also change brain electrical activity. Slow breathing, for example, results in synchrony of brain waves, allowing an integration of different brain regions so they can communicate more effectively.

We also know that our heartbeat speeds up as we inhale and slows down as we exhale, so breathing in a specific pattern also allows us to send signals from the heart that let the brain know we're okay and not in danger. When we increase our HRV using the resources you'll learn in this book, we can return to our window of tolerance. Because of this, consciously changing how we breathe can play a big role in strengthening that all-important vagal brake and improving vagal efficiency.

Although it's normally happening outside of our awareness, changing our breathing to up-regulate or down-regulate our nervous system enhances HRV and vagal tone. It can also bring us back within our window during times of acute or chronic stress, or help us mobilise energy when we need to perform under pressure. Research indicates that practising daily breathing resources designed to increase HRV can decrease stress, anxiety, depression and anger.

Changing the breath in certain ways uses body-up signals to bring about regulation by integrating the thinking brain and survival brain. By altering the type, rate and ratio of breath, we engage the vagal pathways that influence the beating of the heart and the messages sent to the brain. In other words, we can influence our psychological states to improve the symptoms of anxiety, depression and PTSD that are associated with our heart rate.

Typically:

- Slower breathing with prolonged exhalation increases vagal activity and can bring us back into our window of tolerance. Matching inhalation and exhalation (as we do at the start of the 2:1 breathing exercise on page 279) helps maintain autonomic balance.

- Rapid, irregular breathing with sharp inhalations or exhalations increases sympathetic activity and can either shift us out of a dorsal vagal state and into our window of tolerance or cultivate more of the hot sympathetic energy, which when kept in check by the vagal brake gives us focus, strength and clarity.

Trauma-informed breathing resources

Before engaging in embodied and experiential learning, which we know is essential for transforming our nervous system, it's important to acknowledge the relationships between breathing and trauma, as this can help us decide if breathing resources are the best tools for us to use when we're extremely dysregulated.

You've probably seen social media posts that claim all we need to do to calm our nervous system is slow down our breathing. This is very popular advice, and if you ask 10 people on the street what the best way to feel calm is, most will probably reply with a variation of 'Sit still and take long, slow deep breaths.'

This is likely because many of us were taught that breathing slowly was the best way to calm down when we were crying or upset as kids. And while slow, full breathing and focusing on the breath can re-regulate us in some circumstances, it's not a blanket treatment for every state or even every person. This is especially true if:

- **We're already stuck in a cold state:** Our bodily systems are already operating slower than normal, so sitting still and breathing in a way that also slows our heart rate down isn't going to bring us back to our centre. If anything, it might pull us deeper into this cold state, particularly if we extend the exhalation to be longer than the inhalation. In this instance, an activating and upregulating breathing exercise might be better for shifting us into our window of tolerance.

- **We have impaired breathing:** Conditions such as chronic obstructive pulmonary disease (COPD), asthma, Long Covid or other respiratory conditions can make regulating our breathing very difficult. In these instances, trying to regulate our breath might trigger panic responses, so another type of resource will likely be a better fit.
- **There's unresolved trauma in our past:** If the negative event we suffered involved us hyperventilating or experiencing frozen or stuck breath, a breathing exercise might feel overwhelming and even elicit responses from that experience.
- **We suffer from persistent pain:** Depending on where our pain is and how breathing affects it, this type of resource might push us further into a cold state and even worsen our pain. In this case, being on the lookout for interoceptive clues about how breathing is influencing our brain will determine whether we should continue or try something different.
- **We feel agitated and panicked:** Even though this type of exercise can be effective for calming us down when we're agitated, if we're already breathing quickly and experiencing shortness of breath, focusing on our breath might send danger cues to our survival brain and increase our panic. And this is exactly the opposite of what we want.

2. Posture

Earlier in this book, we explored how the proprioceptive system (our sixth sense) helps us avoid danger by keeping us balanced and orienting us in space. Like all our other systems, however, it can learn 'incorrect' lessons that lead to faulty neuroception. Specifically, memories or experiences we may have repressed in our brains can be stored in our reflexive postures and movement patterns. Again, we're not talking about our posture in terms of standing up straight with our shoulders back, but getting to know the reflexive ways our body braces or collapses when we face adversity. In other words, how our bodies move in response to trauma and stress, particularly the ways we're not even conscious of.

Take Lisa, whom we met on page 16, for example. Her body learned to tense up and adopt a protective hunched posture around a certain type of man. The story her body was carrying from her childhood continued to impact her physically and psychologically without her being aware of it.

When we learn to speak the language of our bodies by engaging our proprioceptive system and taking note of its relationship to our body posture, we can start to uncover what it has learned implicitly and how that influences our brain's predictions. Several of the tools we'll learn relate to posture, because how we hold ourselves can shape our thoughts, not to mention our emotional and psychological health.

If you haven't had experience with postural exercises before, you might be surprised to discover how influential they can be. But if you think back to the four fact-finding networks gathering information for our brain, you'll recall that two of them (the proprioceptive and vestibular systems) send constant updates to our brain about how balanced we are, and where our body parts are in space. The way we hold ourselves and how tense or relaxed we are feed into the messages our brain receives about how safe or threatened we are. Through tuning in to our posture, then consciously moving or holding ourselves in certain ways that send body-up signals of safety, we can build regulation and resilience, and start to see ourselves (and heal ourselves) in an integrated way.

3. Containment (tapping or touch) 

Containment resources can help us reconnect with the present moment and our body, especially if we're stuck in a colder state where we feel disconnected or trapped in a loop of rumination. These types of resources are based on the idea that the body is a container that holds everything we experience, including our emotions, thoughts, sensations, memories, and even hopes and dreams. When we tap or touch ourselves to increase sensory input, we can sense this physical container of the body and reconnect with it.

Touching or tapping certain parts of our body can shift our focus from the racing thoughts and worries in our head to the physical sensations we're experiencing. The same way a tight swaddle can calm a distressed baby, hugging yourself tightly can elicit feelings of safety that remind your brain it's not in danger and can help anchor it in the safety of the present moment, regulating your nervous system in the process. It also helps to keep key areas of the brain 'online' when we're moving into dissociation, such as the insula and the Broca's area.

4. Co-regulation

Co-regulation (see page 159) is a powerful tool that requires very little thought. Being around people (or even animals) who are in a calm state is a quick way to modulate our survival brain without necessarily engaging our cognitive thinking brain. These signals bypass the thinking brain, giving us access to emotional regulation even when we're stressed, overwhelmed or our thoughts are chaotic and hard to make sense of.

When our survival brain picks up cues of safety from those around us, we can quickly shift back into our window of tolerance, in much the same way as wild herding animals. If an antelope that outruns a lion is able to rejoin its herd, the calm energy of the herd will regulate it enough that it can shift its body out of survival mode and continue grazing.

Finding the right tool for right now

You now know how important it is to find the right tool for your current state. These two steps will get you started.

Step 1: Take your temperature

Since you can't prescribe an effective treatment unless you know *what* you're treating, your first task is to identify which state you're currently in by tuning in to your internal sensations and signals using your interoception skills. Without the crucial information gathered in these moments of tuning in, we might choose the wrong tool and end up feeling worse.

Each of us needs to develop our own interoceptive practices and make them a regular part of our routine. My own interoceptive practice is now so integrated into my daily routine that it's become as automatic as brushing my teeth. While getting ready in the morning and washing my face, I take an inventory of how I'm feeling and observe any thoughts and sensations that are coming up for me.

All up, listening to what my body is telling me probably takes less than a minute, but checking in with myself a few times daily goes a long way to helping me nip any moments of dysregulation in the bud. If, for example, I notice that I'm feeling tired despite having had lots of sleep the night before, I might make a point of going for a brisk walk during lunch or calling a friend for a chat, because I know those two things boost my mood and give me energy.

Regularly taking my 'temperature' in this way has also made me much better at noticing when I'm starting to feel activated. Instead of letting myself remain tense or irritated, as I would have done in the past, I'll engage a regulating tool to bring myself back to the moment. I've used these tools so many times that they're almost instinctive now – my brain has linked those feelings of tension and fear with the use of calming tools. During a tense meeting, if I notice that my shoulders have raised slightly, I might relax my spine gently against the back of my chair and feel my way into the sensations along my spine, or direct my focus to noticing the solidity of the floor under my feet.

Nobody in the room with me would notice these small, subtle actions, but by redirecting my focus to *exteroceptive* sensations for even a few seconds, the tension in my body often evaporates so that I can re-enter my window of tolerance and think more clearly. When we learn to respond to stressors in new ways, and these become hardwired, we can catch ourselves (a lot of the time, anyway) before straying too far outside that window. This is the beauty of training our nervous system.

Develop emotional granularity

We can influence our body-up and brain-down signals by using something called 'interoceptive selective attention', which is a fancy way of saying that we're not just going to pay attention to our bodily signals, we're going to notice them in a refined, granular way. This links back to that element of specificity. When we can be more specific about the sensations we're experiencing, we can start to uncouple them from the broader emotion or thought that's overwhelming us. This can change the interoceptive network in our brain, particularly between the insula and the amygdala (see pages 92–4).

We know that it takes two or more bodily signals to create an emotion – that's why it's important to understand that interoceptive awareness is not just conscious awareness of these signals and sensations, it's also the ability to describe them. You don't need to explain them to others, you just need to be able to interpret and make sense of your sensations in a detailed and accurate way so you can self-regulate and actively manage your emotions and nervous system responses.

For example, describing the way you feel as 'unwell' is vague and broad. By getting granular, you might be able to identify the signals that are making up that feeling. Your stomach might be tight or gurgling, you might have a rising sensation of bile in your throat. Or perhaps your skin feels cold and clammy and your bones feel achy.

If you say you're hungry, you might also be experiencing tightness and gurgling in your stomach, but these sensations feel very different from those that make you feel unwell. You may also notice that there's tension in your muscles and body because you're starting to get 'hangry'.

To get granular, practise going deeper than a one-word description. If you feel 'anxious', try listing every bodily signal contributing to that feeling. You might realise that you have a lump in your throat or that your breathing is shallow and restricted, and your chest feels tight.

Being able to get granular in this way benefits us in so many ways. To illustrate this, let's look at two examples:

1. After having dinner with a friend, you feel 'bad' or 'off', but you're not sure why. Without more information to go on, you chalk it up to a weird mood and move on, though you still don't feel great about yourself. Later in the week, you realise that your friend hasn't been returning your texts, and this bothers you. You start worrying that you've done something wrong and you're not sure what to do.
2. After having dinner with a friend, you feel guilty. You recognise the emotion because you're familiar with the sensations that usually accompany your feelings of guilt – flushed face, sweaty palms. As you sit with this feeling, you realise that you said something hurtful, and you know your friend was upset by this. When you get home, you call your friend and apologise. She accepts your apology and you speak for a few minutes. After this, you feel relieved and that guilty feeling diminishes, then disappears completely. You're back within your regulated state, and have

also ensured that your friend is no longer upset. It's water under the bridge.

In the second example, you've labelled your feelings with a high degree of specificity, and that means you've been able to deal with the situation effectively. Our bodily signals are the building blocks for *emotional granularity*, which is the ability to experience emotions in a precise and context-specific manner. It's what allows us to recognise what state of our nervous system we have moved into and what may be driving our behaviours.

Neuroscientist and psychologist Lisa Feldman Barrett coined 'emotional granularity' to describe our ability to get specific about our emotional experience. She describes it as our ability to understand and differentiate specific emotions. People with high emotional granularity are better at regulating and coping with stress and other negative emotions, while those with low emotional granularity are less successful in downregulating their negative emotions. Emotional differentiation leads to a better understanding of ourselves and more accuracy when coping with challenges.

This descriptive process comes naturally to some people, while others rely on broader emotional strokes. For example, when describing our emotional state, many of us use vague words and say things like, 'I feel stressed' or 'I'm so angry' or 'That makes me sad.' While these are useful starting points, the more specific we can be, the easier it becomes to modulate our emotions instead of reacting to them. If we investigate a vague feeling such as anger, for example, we're likely to find that we get 'angry' at lots of different things and situations.

Sometimes, anger (which is a hotter response) might be covering for embarrassment, shame or pain (which are emotions we feel when we're in the colder state). Separating this type of 'anger' from the type we feel when someone breaks in to our car is important, because if we try to cope with shame the same way we cope with annoyance, our response won't be appropriate for the situation and it won't soothe our nervous system. Emotions are there to help us decide what wise action we can take next, and the better we are at understanding them, the easier it becomes to meet our needs and make confident decisions. This creates a positive trajectory where we feel empowered and have agency – this is the opposite to what it feels like when we're dysregulated.

Emotion wheel

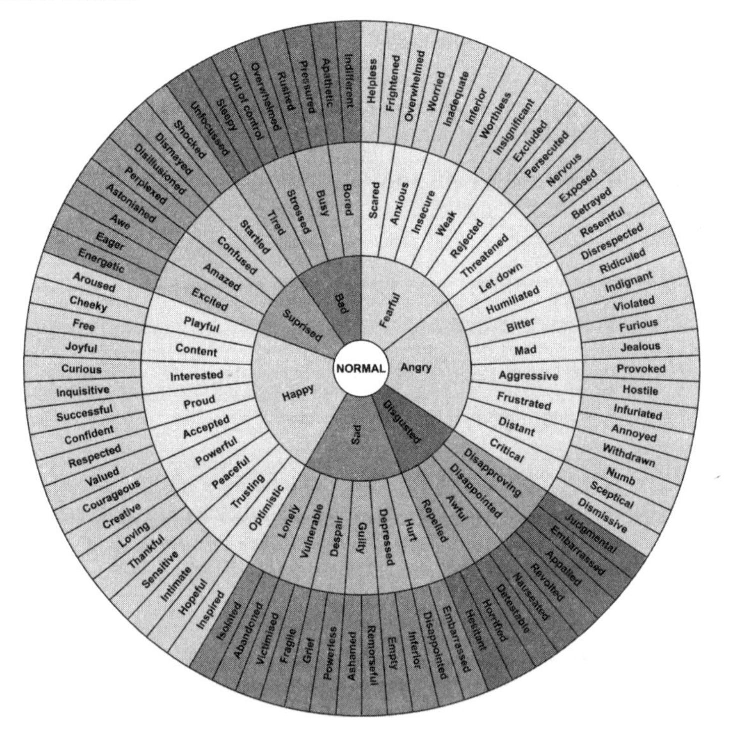

The next time you feel something unpleasant or painful, use this emotion wheel to help you get more specific about what it is you are feeling. If you're 'down', go deeper: are you feeling bored, busy, stressed or tired? Once you identify the next feeling, drill down again. If you said 'bored', then are you feeling apathetic or indifferent? If you said 'lonely', is that because you are feeling isolated or abandoned?

Exercise: Feel, *then* interpret

1. Describe how you're feeling

This exercise is one of my favourites for improving interoceptive accuracy. It's simple, yet very powerful – it may take practise to build this accuracy but just like any skill it's something you can learn.

First, I invite you to write in your notebook or journal how you're feeling *without* using words that describe emotions. Take your time and try to describe how you feel by referring to your internal bodily sensations.

For example, if you're feeling tired, instead of writing that word down, see if you can identify the parts of your body that are sending the signals that you're interpreting as tiredness. If your eyes feel droopy, your body feels heavy or you keep yawning, write those things down.

2. Identify your emotions

Once you've determined the specific signals your body is sending as information, read over your list and use those clues to steer you towards the emotions you are feeling. If your throat and chest feels tight and your hands feel clammy, what emotion do you typically associate with those feelings? Is that how you're feeling now?

Now, I'm going to ask you: *What emotion does this represent?*

To download a worksheet for this process visit www.jessicamaguire.com/emotionalgranularity.

Interoception: Tuning in to your state

Attuning to the sensations in our body enables us to move from *prediction* to *present moment*, and this is one of the best ways to retrain our interoception system, achieve emotional regulation, and build nervous system capacity. Since even complex emotions begin as sensations in the body, turning our attention to those sensations, containing them and then tracking them as they change is the antidote to distress. Our experiences to date have trained our brain–body system to pair certain bodily sensations with certain implicit memories, thoughts and stories. Uncoupling them allows us to look at the sensation more objectively, diffusing highly charged emotions as well as physical pain, and helping transform them fluidly into sensation-based feelings.

First, identify the state you're in so you can use the appropriate interoceptive exercise. For a reminder of how that state feels for you, revisit the map and other notes you made in Chapter 7.

As I've said a few times now, our nervous system loves choice, so having options at your fingertips when selecting resources can make re-regulating ourselves much easier. 'If . . . then' statements can really help with this.

For example, before trying these interoceptive exercises, you might say things like:

- If *I feel overwhelmed when I practise interoception*, then *I'll open my eyes.*
- If *I feel spacey, vague or disconnected from my body while I'm doing this*, then *I'll get up and move around.*
- If *I notice that I'm getting more anxious*, then *I'll stop what I'm doing and try an exteroception exercise instead.*

Write some of your own 'if . . . then' statements in your notebook or journal now, so you can put yourself back in the driver's seat of your nervous system.

If you practise interoception and you notice that you become more dysregulated, you can adapt your training as mentioned above, by using the resources mentioned in the previous chapters to ground you, and by using co-regulation to support you.

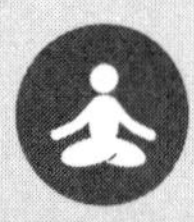

Exercise: Tune in to your too hot state

1. Get comfortable

Begin in a comfortable seated position. You can choose to close your eyes or soften and lower your gaze to allow your attention to travel inward. Follow your breath down into your chest and let your attention settle there, in the space between your breastbone and your spine.

2. Become aware of the sensations in your chest

- What sensations do you notice in this area? Note them mentally or say them quietly to yourself.
- Does it feel easy or difficult to connect with your bodily signals here?

- Does the left side of your body feel the same as the right side?

3. Pay attention to those sensations

See if it's possible to pay attention to the sensations that feel neutral or comfortable and that are easy to connect with.

- Do these sensations move and change?
- Can you notice sensations just as they are – even if they are uncomfortable?

If, on the other hand, a sensation feels unpleasant, you can place one hand over the part it seems to be originating from. Imagine warmth and care travelling from your hand, inward to that vulnerable place inside you. Notice how these sensations change as you pay attention to them.

You may be tempted to get lost in thought with a story about what the sensations mean, but try not to get swept away by that. Can you allow the sensation to be and attend to it without attaching a story to it?

4. Note any changes

Do you notice a change in any of the sensations of activation you felt at the beginning of this exercise? If you're moving closer to your window of tolerance, you may notice your emotions feel less charged, and that your sensations are moving to different parts of your body or becoming different sensations altogether.

Other signs that stress is being discharged and the body is settling include:

- sighing or yawning
- changes in breathing
- bodily sensations in the belly, such as a comfortable gurgling
- muscle tension starting to soften

- thoughts quieting or slowing down
- heat shifting away from the chest
- perhaps even the need to laugh, cry, twist or shake.

5. Pay attention to your belly

Once you notice that the sensations you were feeling when activated have changed, shift your awareness to the belly region and notice the sensations between your belly button and your spine.

- What are they?
- Is it possible to name them?
- Can you notice the sensations just as they are, even if they're uncomfortable?

If a sensation feels unpleasant, place one hand on it and imagine warmth and care travelling from your hand, inward to the vulnerable place inside you. Notice how your sensations change as you pay attention to them.

You may be tempted to get lost in a story about what the sensations mean, but try not to do this. Can you stay connected to the present?

Sometimes, simply tuning in with an interoceptive exercise like this is enough to shift us back into the middle of our window of tolerance. If that's the case for you, congratulations! You've just regulated your nervous system. If, however, focusing on your internal state has increased your dysregulation, turn to Chapter 9, where you'll find a toolkit of bioplasticity resources to help you shift out of this state.

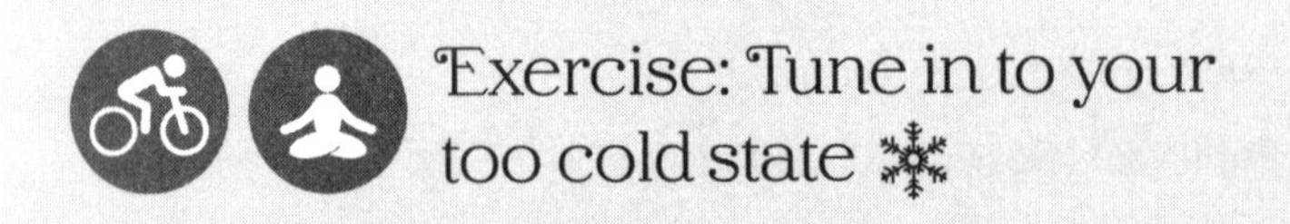

Exercise: Tune in to your too cold state

1. Get comfortable

Begin in a comfortable seated position. You can choose to close your eyes or soften and lower your gaze to allow your attention to travel inward. If you find it hard to connect to your body, gently press your spine into the back of the chair to increase sensory input to your brain – this can help to turn the volume up to integrate important brain regions like the insula. If you still feel numb, make a loose fist and gently tap your chest. This biofeedback is useful if sensations are too small. Follow your breath down into your chest and let your attention land in the space between your breastbone and the spine.

2. Become aware of the sensations in your chest

- What sensations do you notice there?
- Does it feel easy or difficult to connect to bodily signals here?
- Does the left side of your body feel the same as the right side?

If you still feel numb or disconnected from this area of your body add some gentle pressure with your spine against the back of the chair again. Gently tap on your chest with a loose fist.

3. Pay attention to those sensations

See if you can pay attention to sensations that feel neutral or comfortable and are easy to connect to.

- What sensations do you notice?
- Do the sensations move and change?
- Do you feel more connected to your body?

4. Note any changes

If you're starting to shift towards your window of tolerance, out of your cold state, you might notice that you can think clearly again. Here are some other signs that you're moving towards nervous system regulation:

- Your breath might become full or spacious, and feel satisfying or less empty and weak.
- You may feel sensations of warmth in your hands, feet, chest or jaw after feeling cold.
- Alternatively, since the dorsal vagal system conserves energy, you may feel your blood shift towards your extremities.
- You may become aware of your digestive system, with burping, comfortable stomach gurgling or increased motility.
- You could find yourself crying or laughing.

If your sensations feel unpleasant, such as shame or hopelessness, you can place a hand on where they seem to originate and imagine warmth and care travelling from your hand, inward to the vulnerable place inside you.

5. Note how your sensations change

Notice how your sensations change as you attend to them.

You may be tempted to disconnect from these sensations, or you may feel yourself become vague. But is it possible for you to allow the sensation to be just as it is, and tune in to it without a story, only with care? If you start to drift into the dorsal vagal state, you could stand up to upregulate your system.

6. Pay attention to your belly

Once the sensations in your chest have changed, can you shift your awareness down into your belly region?

- Can you notice any sensations between your belly button and your spine? If you feel numb or disconnected, you could lightly stroke the skin of your belly and then let your attention travel inward.
- What sensations are here?
- Is it possible to name them?
- Can you notice those sensations just as they are – even if they're uncomfortable?

If a sensation feels unpleasant, you can place a hand on it and imagine warmth and care travelling from your hand to the vulnerable place inside you.

Notice how sensations change as you attune to them. You may observe that the sensations that you identified from the dorsal vagal state begin to change as your sympathetic state kicks into action. You may notice more energy in your sensations, more movement or even different sensations. If you still feel vague or disconnected, you could gently press your feet into the floor.

If you shifted more to the middle of your window of tolerance, then you re-regulated your nervous system. You might experience this discharge of stress activation as your body settling, sighing or yawning. You may also notice your body twitching or shaking. Muscle tension in your body will start to soften. You may notice that you can think clearly again, as if a fog has lifted from between you and the room you're in.

Standing increases your heart rate and provides more proprioceptive and interoceptive information that will activate important brain regions that can go offline when you dissociate form your body.

Light touch has been shown to activate a specialised group of skin receptors that communicate with the insula – this is a great intervention if you find it challenging to connect to sensations.

If your dysregulation has increased, turn to Chapter 10 for exercises that can help.

Anchoring in the just-right state

When you're already in, or have found your way back to your set point, there are several ways that you can settle into or 'anchor' in this state. This is beneficial because it prolongs the amount of time you spend feeling balanced and regulated

The vagal brake: establishing your natural set point

In Chapter 5, we discussed the crucial role the vagal brake plays in nervous system regulation. When we can engage or release the vagal brake in line with the demands being placed on us and shift easily between all of the states, we have what's called good vagal efficiency.

You can train your vagal brake and increase vagal efficiency through breathing resources that increase HRV, but first you need to record a baseline so you know what your natural heart rate and breathing pattern look like when you're calm and regulated. If you're currently feeling calm, sociable and at ease, this is a good time to find your baseline and establish that natural set point.

Think about the pace of your heart.

- Does it feel like it's pumping at a 'regular' speed? You may not be able to notice it if you're regulated.

- Does your heart rate feel stable?
- Are your breaths full and easy?
- Are your thoughts manageable and not overwhelming?
- If you're wearing a smartwatch with a heart monitor, what reading did that give you?

I encourage you to write down all of the answers to these questions in your notebook or journal so that you can refer back to them while practising the breathing exercises in Chapters 9 and 10.

Movement

When we want to anchor in the ventral vagal state, movement can help us feel safe, accepted and at ease. Anything that makes you feel at home in yourself, such as gardening, hiking with friends or doing a calming yoga class, ticks this box. In this state, we have full access to our social engagement system, and can regulate and connect with others.

Ventral vagal: What prolongs the experience or anchors you here?	
Low energy	**High energy**
Stroll on the beach	Gentle walk
Playing with children	Gardening
Tai Chi	Hiking with friends
Team sports with others	Yoga/Pilates
	Swim

Reflect back on a time you were in this state. What activities might you engage in to keep yourself feeling sociable and content? Write them down on in your notebook or journal.

If movement is challenging for you because of persistent pain, imagining or visualising movement can help sharpen your sensory map and influence your neuroimmune system in a positive way.

Music

If you've ever listened to a fast-paced song while preparing to play in a soccer or football game, or during a spin class, you already know that music can help us shift states. And if we're within our window of tolerance, it can also help us anchor there. This is likely because training the middle ear muscles improves our neuroception, which helps us to tune in to cues of safety instead of cues of threat.

Sound therapy has been shown to be an effective tool for improving self-regulation and thus making social engagement more accessible. In one study, it was associated with increased HRV, which indicates improvement in vagal tone. Music, at particular frequencies, works directly on our middle ear muscles and autonomic nervous system, enhancing the function of the cranial nerves (some of which work interdependently with the vagus nerve to activate our social engagement system). Music can, therefore, be an important tool for retraining our nervous system. Listening to music that makes you feel calm, centred and content will have a similar effect, and help you anchor in your just-right state.

In order to better understand how listening to music impacts you physically and emotionally, I invite you to make your own playlist for each of your states. It's just as important to find music that anchors us in our calmest, most connected and most sociable state as it is to find music that amps us up or calms us down.

Imagine seeing a good friend and feeling connected with them. What five songs or pieces would you want to listen to during or after this meet-up? Write them down in your notebook or journal so you can remember what to add to your playlist.

In each state – particularly in the dorsal vagal state and the sympathetic nervous system state – it's important to listen to music that makes us feel safe. Safe to be anchored in a state, and safe to move freely between states as we find appropriate. Like so much of the bioplasticity training we've discussed so far in the book, music is a tool we can use to build resilience, and to lead a fuller, more contented life in which we feel autonomous.

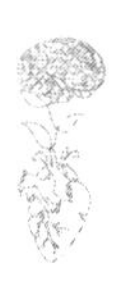

Now that you know where you're at now and how to approach your nervous system reset, it's time for the nuts and bolts of the book – the toolsets you need to find your ideal set point and stay there.

9

Toolkit for shifting out of your too hot state

As we've seen throughout the book, our vagus nerve plays an integral role in almost all of our bodily functions and has a huge impact on our nervous system, behaviours, emotions and thoughts. Now that we know so much more about the physiology of our many systems and how interconnected they are, it's time to practise training these systems with the tools best suited to our current state. If you determine that you're in a hotter state, the tools in this chapter should bring your nervous system back to a state of calm sociability.

A few of these tools can be practised in moments of extreme stress, too. The better you get at noticing when you're shifting into an activated state and remembering to use these tools, the more you'll find them start to become instinctive. Training will bring about bioplasticity, and your body–brain system will link the actions involved in those body-up tools to feelings of activation.

That's been my experience, at least, and I notice myself slipping into breathing or grounding exercises automatically when I find myself in a challenging or heated situation. Within a minute,

I'm usually back within my window of tolerance and able to think rationally. When we can recover from stress and even traumatic events appropriately over the course of our lives, we become so much more emotionally resilient, not to mention healthier physically and mentally.

Let's revisit the metaphor we used earlier in the book, where the messages whizzing around the body are planes flying in and out of different airports with one central airport connecting many flights – the insula. If we're triggered by something but we can send signals of safety to our survival brain by using the bottom-up tools in these chapters, we have the power to change the 'planes' it deploys in response.

As the new planes we've sent by practising these tools land at the survival brain airport with their messages of safety, connecting flights carry this message to the main airport, which we said was like Heathrow (the insula). The planes that were about to take off carrying orders to jump to high alert are suddenly grounded. Instead, new planes carrying orders to maintain homeostasis taxi out onto the runway and take off instead.

As you already know, in this state, your heart is likely to be beating faster, you might have racing thoughts, and you likely have a bit of energy – or a lot – that you'd like to release from the body. There are several ways of doing this. To start, I recommend working through the tools that follow one by one – there's a method to their order, and it will help you build capacity over time. If you tend to feel anxious or dysregulated when you notice bodily signals or your breath, start with the tools in chapters 9 and 10 first, to bring regulation and also tune in to the sensations outside your body (exteroception). This is a trauma-informed way to practise. The table below gives an indication of the tools that can be applied to varying degrees of activation.

Choosing tools for the hot state 

What do I feel tuning in to my nervous system?	What led me here?	What tools or strategies will shift me out of here?
Anger, tension, heat. I can't sit still. My thoughts are going round and round.	I read the comments section on social media where someone argued with me.	Shaking (page 252) 1:2 breathing (page 255) Talking to a friend Setting limits on social media
Scared and anxious. I can't sit still. My thoughts are telling me I'm going to fail and things will fall apart.	I was given extra tasks at work and my child needs help with a project too. The house feels disorganised. I can't keep up.	Movement resources (page 250) Music playlist (page 264) Making a list of tasks and delegating
Heat and tension in my chest. My heart is beating fast. I feel a fear of rejection like I used to when my dad didn't show up.	Someone I've recently started dating hasn't texted me back.	Music playlist (page 264) Touch exercise (page 259) Calling a friend to go for a walk

Bioplasticity tools

Posture tools

Working with your body's posture is such a simple way to change the integration of the brain–body system. Changing the way our body is positioned against gravity influences our blood pressure, which in turn influences our autonomic state.

The baroreceptors (pressure sensors) near the heart (see page 113) are there to help the body maintain blood pressure at a relatively constant level, especially when we change body position. This is important to keep blood pumping consistently up to the brain when we move from lying down to standing up. Stretching of baroreceptors as a result of increased blood pressure will create a shift in the activity of the vagus nerve, leading to a change in heart rate and blood pressure to bring the system back to homeostasis.

When you're feeling keyed up in this hotter state and want to get back to your just-right state, you may benefit from lying down on your back. Blood pressure is at its lowest when we're in this position, and our heart can easily pump blood to the brain because it's not working against gravity as it would when we're standing. This automatically lowers our blood pressure, slowing our heart rate and breathing.

Let's return to Laura, whom we met back in Chapter 1. She was anxious about going to a party for days beforehand, and went into the event in a 'flight' state. Consequently, her body language and posture at the party were tense, and the rigidity of her posture only sent more cues of danger and stress to her brain, feeding her hot state and reinforcing the narrative she was telling herself, which was that she'd feel awkward and have trouble connecting and relaxing.

Even though Laura intellectually wanted to go to the party and meet new people, her body was preventing her from relaxing enough to enjoy herself and form genuine connections by accessing the social engagement system. If she can't develop the autonomic awareness to realise how her body is influencing her experiences, Laura will remain in this state, and these stories about herself will follow her wherever she goes.

The following exercise uses sensory information from the exteroceptors, proprioceptors and vestibular system, so it can be a powerful way to regulate ourselves while engaging the vagus nerve and building vagal tone.

Tool 1: Using posture to downregulate

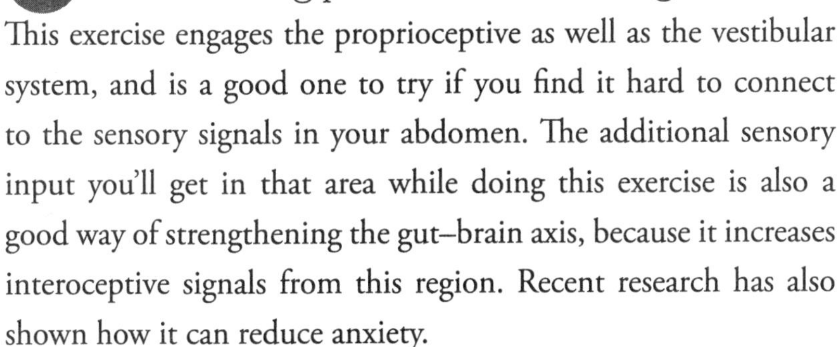

This exercise engages the proprioceptive as well as the vestibular system, and is a good one to try if you find it hard to connect to the sensory signals in your abdomen. The additional sensory input you'll get in that area while doing this exercise is also a good way of strengthening the gut–brain axis, because it increases interoceptive signals from this region. Recent research has also shown how it can reduce anxiety.

Before you start: You'll need a yoga mat (or something similar to lie on), a blanket (similar in size to a yoga blanket) or throw and two large pillows or a yoga block.

1. Get into a seated kneeling position at the bottom of your mat with your buttocks resting on your heels.
2. Place the yoga block or stacked pillows in front of you nearer the top of the mat.
3. 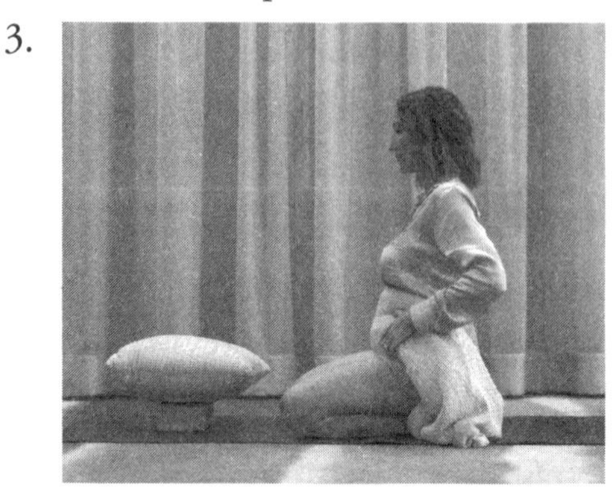
Fold the blanket in half, and then half again. Place it against your stomach, under your rib cage and above your hips. (You may need to adjust the position as you go and how many folds you'll require as you add pressure.) Put your hands in front of you and slowly walk them forward – the blanket should add gentle pressure to your abdomen. If you need to widen your knees, feel free.
4. 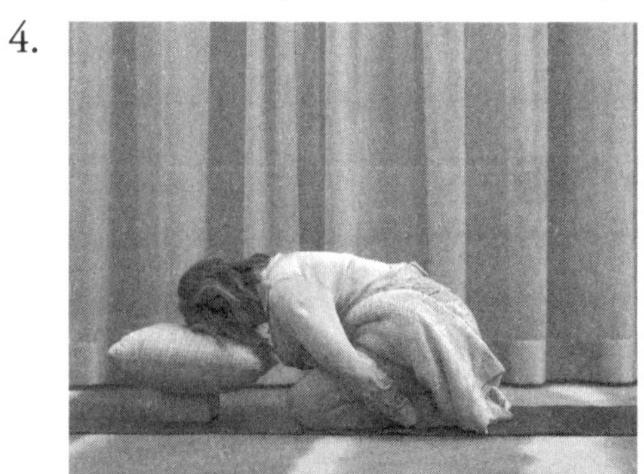
Next, rest your forehead on your yoga block or two pillows, so the pressure is distributed over your brow bone. If this is uncomfortable or you have knee pain, you can rest your arms on a large therapy ball in front of you rather than lay your head on the block or pillows.

You should feel firm pressure from the blanket on your abdominal region, but it shouldn't be painful (if it is, you can unfold the blanket a little so it's not as thick). You can keep your eyes open or close them to help you connect to your body, or simply soften your gaze on the floor and bring your attention to your body.

5. Take a snapshot of your nervous system now before you get started on the rest of the exercise. Where is your nervous system thermostat currently set? Begin by noticing the points of your body that are connected to your environment:
   - Feel your legs connected to the floor and the difference between the left and right side of your pelvis and your right and left leg.
   - Notice areas of pressure from the parts of your belly touching the blanket.
   - Notice your arms and hands connecting to the ground.
   - Notice any pressure on your skin, even the pressure of your clothing.
   - Notice the pressure over your brow bone and the sensations that brings.

   Now bring your attention to your feet and lower legs on the floor. Although your attention may drift to other things in the room, see if you can, for a moment, focus on the exteroceptive signals from the tactile input of your body making contact with your environment.

   Bring your awareness to your pelvis. Can you gently rock your weight to the left side, noticing how your trunk shifts over with you? Feel the difference in pressure through your left leg.

   Return to the centre. Next, allow your weight to rock onto the right leg, feeling the left side of your pelvis lift, and let your weight shift over as your trunk follows.

You may notice how the weight shifts in your arms and also on your face.

Continue to slowly move side to side, finding a rhythm that's comfortable and enjoyable, noting how that attunes you to your nervous system. You might make the movements smaller and faster. You might make them slower and bigger. Just like a parent might rock a baby, imagine you could rock to settle and soothe your own nervous system.

Continue to bring your attention to your feet and the legs, taking in this exteroceptive information.

6. Move back to your original kneeling position and notice your hands resting on your lap or one on the other, and take in that exteroceptive information. There might be areas that are easy to feel and connect with on your skin. Bring your hands together and gently press them into each other, noticing the sensory information on your skin.

   Finally, bring the hands to the outside of your knees. Can you gently press your hands into the outside of the legs without letting the legs move? This isometric contraction allows sensory information from your proprioceptors to give input to the brain. You could let that relax and slowly repeat the pressure three or four more times, again noticing what happens in your brain–body system.

Has this downregulation exercise helped regulate you?

When you feel ready, return to stillness and take a snapshot of your brain–body system now.

- What does your body feel like?
- Do you feel more 'in' your body?

- What sensations do you notice?
- What is your breath like?
- What urges or impulses come to mind?
- What thoughts do you notice?
- Do you feel more present 'in' your mind?
- How has your nervous system thermostat changed?

Tool 2: Exteroceptive exercises for those 10/10 stress moments 🚹

Even though how well we manage our emotions will be influenced by how good we are at recognising and accurately labelling our internal bodily signals, if we're experiencing a 10/10 level of stress arousal, tuning in and using interoception will generally be unpleasant and overwhelming. When we're dysregulated or experiencing panic, we often define our reality based on signals from our interoceptors (what's going on inside us), and at these times they can be overwhelming: a pounding heart, a churning gut, or a feeling like we can't breathe. Focusing on those even more won't do much to bring us back towards regulation.

In these cases, exteroceptive practices that focus attention on the signals coming from outside of ourselves (e.g. sights, sounds, smells) are often much more effective.

If I'm feeling really scared and my heart is racing and I'm dizzy, I might conclude (or neurocept) that my external environment is dangerous. But if I pause and use my exteroceptive senses to take in what's actually going on in my external environment, I can better discern whether I'm safe or not.

Here's an example scenario for what using your exteroceptive senses might look like.

You've walked to a cafe because you had an argument with your partner and you stormed off. Now you're starting to panic that they might move out and break up with you. You notice your heart racing and breathing rate increasing, and you even feel dizzy. After ordering, you sit down in the corner. You remember that using your exteroceptive senses might be helpful in moments like this; you move your eyes to orient yourself in your environment, which helps to re-engage the vagal brake and can bring you back inside the window of tolerance; and you then start to mentally itemise everything you observe in your immediate surroundings: *The woman across from me is wearing a pink scarf. The coffee cup in my hands is warm. The air in this cafe smells like hot chocolate. There's jazz playing on the stereo . . .*

After a few minutes of this, you feel calm enough to text your partner and extend an olive branch.

Stress indicator

Because the vagus nerve is deeply involved with *both* the social engagement system and how we cope with and recover from stress, one important indication that we're having difficulties managing our stress arousal is that we'll have trouble maintaining supportive and satisfying relationships. This can show up in our personal and professional relationships.

Movement-based tools

In the sympathetic nervous system state, the mind and body are in a state of hyperarousal. We might feel anxious, concerned, irritated or even angry. Our body feels tight and constricted. Whether consciously or unconsciously, our jaw might be clenched, and we might feel a sensation to run or feel like we can't sit still. And our thoughts become fear-focused. When we're in this state, we need to discharge the excess energy that's been activated and is sitting in our nervous system. The sympathetic system is a mobilising system that brings energy into your body to make you take action (fight or flight). This is a good thing when we need to take on challenges to rise to the occasion. But this mobilisation can feel like anxiety when it continues to build.

Movement resources can help us discharge this pent-up stress – often fairly quickly. Much like a duck, after it's squabbled with another duck, discharges that energy by flapping its wings, we can shake our limbs slightly, or even vigorously. This can help us expel the pent-up energy being generated by being stuck in the sympathetic state. How much movement you need to successfully bring you back to regulation depends on where you are on the activation scale below.

Sympathetic: How to use mobilisation energy in organised and safe ways	
Low energy	**High energy**
Use fidgets	Seated shaking
Go outside and move	Do a spin class
Go to yoga with a friend	Dancing
Get up and walk	Standing shaking
	Jogging
	Swimming

If, for example, there's a bit of sympathetic activation going on in our body but it's relatively low, light movement such as going for a walk or even vacuuming the house might be enough to discharge that feeling. If, on the other hand, we have lots of sympathetic activation – perhaps we feel anxious or really antsy – a more rigorous activity such as running or swimming, or even shaking (see the following exercise) will be required to discharge some of that activation.

Let's use Laura's experience at the party from Chapter 1 as an example of when movement might be a useful regulation tool. Before the party, she was feeling incredibly anxious. On the way there, she noticed that her palms felt sweaty and her heart was racing. If you feel comfortable doing so, reflect on a time when you felt this way about an event. It doesn't have to be a party, just any event that made you feel similarly anxious. Now consider what movement your body might have been urging you to do in that moment. What movement could you have done to discharge that energy? List five of these in your notebook or journal.

Had Laura decided to go for a short run or a swim before getting ready for the party, she would likely have been able to release quite a bit of that pent-up anxiety and reconnect her to her body.

Tool 3: Shaking

If vigorous movement is called for and you can't set aside time for a block of exercise, a few minutes of shaking can be a great way to discharge energy. This exercise is as simple as the name suggests. Depending on how you're feeling and how many people are around you, this can involve just shaking your hands up and down, or your arms, legs or full body if needed.

You may find that small movements help you attune to how you're feeling. If you notice anger or big emotions, you may find that bigger movements and an elevation of your heart rate allow a discharge of that stress activation.

1. Start in a standing position with your feet hip-width apart. It's helpful if you have enough room around you to spread out your arms.
2. Notice your feet on the floor and your arms by your sides, then bend your elbows and start shaking through your hands. You can start small or big – notice how your body wants to move.
3. Raise your arms and shake them both, working up to a speed where your heart rate increases. If you feel the need, you could try shaking one arm at a time, or continue with both.
4. Notice what happens to your bodily sensations, your emotions and your thoughts as you shake.
5. If you'd like, you can shake one foot as well. Then the other, if you like. You can do this – either lightly or vigorously – for a few moments.
6. Notice what's happening to the sensations in your body.
    - Do you feel a sense of relief?
    - Is there a bit more spaciousness in your chest and mind?
    - Is your body starting to relinquish those feelings of tightness and restriction?

Has shaking helped regulate you?

Now come into a seated posture that supports you and reflect on the following questions:

- Does your breath feel more spacious or does it feel easier to breathe?

- Has the tension in your body eased?
- If there was tension in your shoulders, has that let go?
- If you were gritting your teeth or clenching your jaw, has that changed? How?
- What's happened to your thoughts? Are any stories still circling in your mind?
- Have your thoughts quietened down or maybe slowed down?
- Do you feel more connected to the present moment?

I recommend taking out your notebook and adding your observations under the heading 'Shaking resource' near your window of tolerance map

Breathing tool

When we're in the sympathetic nervous system state, the number of breaths we take per minute is usually higher than our average inhalations and exhalations. The vagal brake, as we've seen, has withdrawn, activating that mobilisation of energy.

In order to shift out of the sympathetic nervous system state, and re-enter our window of tolerance, we can begin by using 1:1 breathing, and from there we can move into 1:2.

Go gently

Remember, there's no one blanket tool for every situation. If you are experiencing high levels of dysregulation or panic, paying attention to the breath where it's difficult to take a deep breath or there's air hunger, may send cues to the survival brain that there is a big threat. Similarly, if breathing is particularly difficult for you, and does, in fact, trigger dysregulation, I encourage you to use some of the other tools. Learning to recognise what state of your nervous system you're in at any given moment and being able to track how it changes as you use breathing resources first, is important. (See 'Trauma-informed breathing resources' on page 219 for more.)

Tool 4: 1:2 breathing

(For an audio recording of this exercise please go to www.jessicamaguire.com/breathe).

1. Start by simply taking note of your breathing wherever it feels the most neutral or pleasant, or easiest. See if you can allow your body to breathe on its own, as it does naturally so many times each day.
2. Now pay attention to your in-breath. How many seconds does it take for you to breathe in?
3. Next pay attention to your out-breath. How many seconds does it take for you to breathe out?
4. Note which is shorter, your in-breath or out-breath.
5. See if you can naturally allow your breath to become full, without creating any tension in neck, shoulders, chest or diaphragm – tensing those muscles can increase sympathetic nervous system activation. Allow your breath to gently and gradually lengthen, prioritising 'softness' in your body muscles.
6. See if you can allow whichever part of your breath was shorter, the in-breath or the out-breath, to lengthen just

one count. Again, relax your body and spend several breaths here, noticing anything that happens in your brain–body system as you do.

7. Now lengthen the shorter part of your breath, until your in-breath and out-breath are equal. It's okay if you pause between each breath or between the inhalation and exhalation. Just allow your body to find a rhythm that's natural and easy as it shifts into a 1:1 breathing pattern.
8. Notice what happens to your body and to your thoughts when you shift into this breathing pattern.
9. Relax your body if necessary, especially your neck and shoulders. Where do you feel your body is mostly breathing? If it's your upper chest and shoulders, can you place your hands on the sides of your lower ribs and imagine each in-breath shifting your ribcage out to the sides? Again, keep the neck and shoulders relaxed. You might try taking five to 10 breaths here, then let your arms rest back down with your hands in your lap.
10. Invite your body to soften and receive the breath so that it's a little bit deeper, keeping a matched in-breath and out-breath. You may find you can get to an inhalation and exhalation of about three seconds each, slowly building up their length while keeping your posture relaxed. There's no need to rush or to try to push yourself to take a deeper breath.
11. If you feel comfortable, you can slowly increase the length of your in-breaths and out-breaths, and continue relaxing in your body. If you're in the sympathetic nervous system state it can be helpful to lengthen each exhalation by one extra count to engage the vagal brake. Notice what happens

when you lengthen your out-breath slightly. Is it possible to invite the breath out to deepen rather than force the exhalation? Continue for a few more breath cycles.

Has 1:2 breathing helped regulate you?

Now that the exercise is over, take note of anything that's changed in your brain–body system.

- What bodily signals do you notice?
- Has your heart rate slowed? If so, does it feel more in line with your normal set point? (Revisit the baseline exercise you did in Chapter 7.)
- Does your breathing feel deeper and less restricted?
- Is there a greater sense of ease in your body?
- What emotions are coming up for you?
- Has your posture relaxed and softened?
- What are your thoughts centred around?

When we regulate our breathing this way and control our breath, we're activating the vagal brake, signalling to our brain that we're not in danger. If we revisit the example of Jenny from Chapter 5, whose worries about her sister and the isolation of the pandemic were keeping her in that hot state, we can imagine how 1:2 breathing might restabilise her.

By breathing with control, and slowing her heart rate down, Jenny could signal to her brain that she's not in danger – despite what her survival brain thinks. She wouldn't have needed to do this all the time, either. As little as 10 minutes a day could give her extended benefits and help shift her from her new set point in that hotter state, and back into her window of tolerance or the ventral vagal state, where she'd feel calm and centred. Over time, she could gradually build up to longer and longer exhalation cycles to train her system further, creating a bioplasticity reset so she could find regulation again.

A breathing technique such as this one will be enough to bring many people back inside their window of tolerance, and back to a sense of calm. For others, though, breathing won't be enough. If you don't find this exercise helpful in your current state, try one of the other bioplasticity tools in this chapter.

Tools for working with the fascia

This tool can actually be used in all of the states, but it's useful for moving out of the too hot state when we're fearful of our pain. One of the resources I recommended to patients to help them connect to their skin, fascia and soft tissue – and build this connection for regulation – focuses on the thoracolumbar fascia, is the large diamond shape on our lower back. This can be useful if you experience persistent pain or if you feel disconnected from your body, especially the gut. It is also useful if you find interoception challenging, because light touch receptors can wake up our interoception. (Reminder: I strongly recommend talking to your healthcare professional if you have any doubts about whether these tools are appropriate for you!)

Tool 5: Touch (partner exercise)

Since this exercise requires a partner, it's a two-for-one in the sense that it engages fascia, and therefore your interoceptive system, *as well as* co-regulation, and therefore your social engagement system. It's hands-on, so you'll want to do this with someone you feel very comfortable with. This exercise can also be great if you tend to dissociate from your body and sensations.

This tool recruits your complex and potentially powerful brain mechanisms to fine-tune the signals that are coming in, and it can sharpen the sensory maps in your brain. You'll recall we talked about the sensory maps and 'smudging' on page 146.

1. Lie on your stomach in a comfortable position. Ask your partner to touch you lightly in random locations on your lower back with either a wine cork or a pen lid. Your task is to identify what tool was used and where exactly you have been touched by pointing there shortly afterwards. You could record your accuracy (measured out of 20) and if you are able to do this daily, record your progress. If your partner can provide feedback as to where they touched your back and correct you – even better.
2. Next, your partner will lightly draw a letter or a number on your back and you will identify it. As above, you can record your accuracy, so you can track your progress with bioplasticity.

Tool 6: Touch (solo exercise)

If you have the tolerance, you can progress to using deep pressure to stimulate other receptors in your proprioceptive system which, as previously noted, has been shown to improve anxiety. Using two soft massage balls or tennis balls wrapped in a sock you're going to train your brain–body system.

1. In order to get in touch with this part of your body I recommend sitting on a full-backed supportive chair,

planting your feet flat on the floor, and seeing where your set point is currently at.

As you connect with your body, see if you can notice sensations in your lower back.

- Are there areas that are easy to connect to?
- Are there areas where it's challenging to notice sensations? Perhaps they feel dull, vague or numb. Try to let go of a story about what that might mean or how things should be.

2. Lightly place the massage or tennis balls between your back and the chair, in the space between your lowest rib and your pelvis. Roll them up and down then side to side, avoiding any bony prominences.
3. Now I invite you to experiment with the pressure. What happens when you press firmer with deep, slow pressure?
4. Continue for several minutes then let your hands rest in your lap. Has the temperature setting on your thermostat shifted at all? Do you feel a difference in how you connect now to the sensations in your lower back compared with before you used this tool?

Tool 7: Deeper pressure for your stretch zone

The fourth and final part of this series progresses to deeper pressure, which involves the proprioceptive and interoceptive systems. This is a wonderful way to 'train' these systems, where imbalances have been associated with anxiety, depression, chronic pain, and IBS and other gastrointestinal issues. You have the ability to modulate the amount of pressure that you apply and to stop whenever you choose.

This exercise can be used to downregulate *and* up-regulate. It's useful for moving out of the hotter sympathetic state because it can increase vagal tone, inhibit all of that sympathetic activation, decrease any bracing or tension in the body, and help regulate breathing, all of which will tell your brain that there's no danger. It's useful to help you shift out of the dorsal vagal state if you have dissociated or have difficulty connecting with it. This will help you keep the insula and frontal lobes 'online'.

I think of the following technique as applying mild to moderate stress to the brain–body system. It's a gentle way of getting into that all-important stretch zone, where real growth takes place. This can help us cultivate the resilience we need to notice and attune to uncomfortable sensations without feeling overwhelmed or being pushed outside our window of tolerance. It's also a way for us to change our brain's predictions about which sensations are threatening or safe.

As you use this tool, the key is to recognise whether you're moving into a hotter state. Signs of this include clammy palms, clenching your jaw, bracing, nausea, and a sense of anxiety or agitation.

If this exercise moves you into the colder dorsal vagal state, you might feel less connected to your body, the room may go fuzzy, and you may feel your energy drop or have a sense of collapse in your body. In any case, it's best to use less pressure and use this resource for a shorter time, or revert back to the two previous trainings.

1. Lie on the floor with your knees bent and slowly roll onto one side. Slide the massage or tennis balls (see Tool 6 on page 259) to the same area you massaged in Tool 6, avoiding any bony landmarks. Slowly return to your back

and allow your weight to sink onto the balls, keeping your knees bent. If the pressure is too much, you can prop pillows under your head as well as each shoulder.

This may feel uncomfortable and take you to the 'edge' of your stretch zone, but that's okay. Remember, we want to introduce some discomfort without moving outside our window of tolerance. If it becomes too much, you can stop at any time by rolling onto one side.

2. As you allow yourself to relax, see what sensations you can notice in your body.
   - What's it like to fix your attention on sensations that may be unpleasant or uncomfortable? You may need to re-relax into your body by softening your jaw and face.
   - Do you notice a change in your internal thermostat?
   - Is there a change in your breathing, or in the sensations and emotions in your body?
3. If you feel like continuing, you can gently lower one side of your pelvis slightly, then the other so that the balls roll side to side. Do you prefer to add this movement or to keep this pressure static? See if you can attune to your body and invite it to soften rather than forcing anything to happen.
4. Practise for as long as you choose to. Once finished, take a reading of your inner thermostat and see if it's changed.

In the dorsal vagal state, this tool increases sensory input into the brain regions that help us to be aware of our sense of self, allowing us to reconnect with our body. If we've been dissociated and are not ready to progress to interoceptive resources yet, this is a great way to train our brain–body system without overwhelming it. Neurodivergent individuals may find this useful if interoception on its own is challenging, particularly if sensations are too 'quiet.'

If you can, I encourage you to try this tool, in any of the states. Consider how this it makes you feel physically and mentally. Notice your breath, your heart rate and the stories that are playing in your head.

Give yourself options!

I know I've said this a few times now, but it bears repeating: the nervous system loves choice, and re-regulating it comes from listening to it and honouring your needs. Dysregulation will always be amplified if you feel powerless and lacking in agency. It's important for you to feel like you have options and some sense of control.

Using 'if . . . then' statements can really help. For example:

1. If *I feel overwhelmed when I practise interoception*, then *I'll open my eyes.*
2. If *I feel spacey or vague*, then *I'll get up and move around.*
3. If *I notice that I'm getting more anxious*, then *I'll go back to my exteroception training.*

Take out your notebook or journal and write some of your own if . . . then statements to put yourself back in the driver's seat of your nervous system.

If at any point you notice that you're becoming more dysregulated, you can adapt your training as mentioned in the statements above, by using the resources mentioned in this chapter to ground you, and by using co-regulation to support you.

Tool 8: Create a playlist to bring you out of your hot state

As we saw in Chapter 8, research tells us that simply listening to music has the power to impact us physically and emotionally, so as I suggested then, consider your own playlist for each nervous system state. In the hotter state, music that is slower paced and calming can help bring us back within our window of tolerance, or any music that attunes to where we're at. That might mean some rock music if we're angry, or some EDM if we're antsy or feeling playful.

Open your notebook or journal and list five songs you think might bring you into a state of calmness after being in a state of hyperarousal. Now that you've chosen the songs, grab your phone and create a playlist of them right now. Add to this playlist whenever you discover a song that you find calming or peaceful. If you could use some downregulating now, pop some headphones on, hit play, close your eyes and let the music bring you back to yourself. Next time you feel yourself getting swept away into this hot state, all you need to do is hit play.

Tool 9: Create a playlist for finding your play state

As we discussed in Chapter 1, sometimes we *want* to stay in this hotter state because it benefits us to have access to that extra energy when we need it. If you are gearing up for a big athletic game, or preparing for a presentation, then you need to be in this upper window in order to reach peak performance.

Imagine these two scenarios, or similar ones relevant to your life, and consider what music you might play to downregulate yourself enough to bring your thinking brain online and calm your systems a little, while also keeping that energetic, animated and motivated state. This is the blended state of play we talked about earlier, and the music that shifts you into this state and keeps you there is likely to be something up tempo that makes you feel excited, happy or like jumping and dancing around.

List five songs that might help you feel playful then add those to your playlist.

Simple tools for co-regulation quick wins

To move away from your hot state and get your social engagement system going, try some of these activities. Make a list of your own ideas in your notebook or journal and add it to whenever you think of another.

Alone (with strangers or animals)	Together (with people you know)
Take yourself (and your dog if you have one) to the park Go for a walk on the beach Do a spin class Do a yin yoga class	Catch a movie with your best friend Do a dance class with your partner Go to a comedy night with your sibling

Now bring in brain-down regulation

Now that we've explored some powerful body-up tools, it's time to bring everything together by introducing some brain-down regulation. As we know, working with the body in isolation is no better than working with the brain in isolation. To successfully reset our nervous system and maintain equilibrium in the future, we must integrate both body-up and brain-down information. We could also look at those things that have an outside-in impact on us and our nervous system. This includes the biological systems in our brain and body, as well as the ones we can't see – those sensations, emotions and thoughts that fuel the never-ending loop of energy inside us. It also includes things such as our relationships, the community we live in and our current work–life balance.

Research tells us that anxiety and depression are characterised by (and possibly even partly *caused* by) our incorrect expectations about the future.

For this reason, when you're back in a comfortable, secure and regulated state, it's well worth investigating the areas of your life where brain-down predictions are occurring and impacting your physiology. Once you know where those predictions and stories live, you can begin to mentally uncouple them from the sensory information you receive in the present moment.

I see this exercise as a sort of treasure hunt, except in this case you're searching for limiting thoughts and stories rather than gold or jewels. It may not be as lucrative but it's equally valuable.

Tool 10: Locate your areas of faulty neuroception

Let's say one of our brain-down expectations is that we'll always be let down in relationships, causing us to pull away from people as soon as they don't reply to our messages and creating a strong fear of abandonment.

When stress arousal is high, the survival brain communicates with us through sensations and emotions that we feel in our body. What might help us first is learning that it's embodied and experiential. Once we've practised enough resources to help us feel anchored in our window of tolerance, we might consider the following questions or lean in to co-regulation with someone we trust, in order help us to get in touch with our bodily sensations and emotions.

By answering these questions, you're guiding yourself to connect experientially with your physiology and integrate the body-up with the brain-down. This is where we can lean into interoception to help cultivate regulation and attune to physical sensations and impulses as they move through our body, and sifting through the thoughts that arise. Try sitting in a way where you can be as comfortable as possible, let your attention shift to your body and ask the following questions:

- How does this fear show up in your body?
- How does it feel to be 'in touch' with your fear?
- If you could pass a microphone to these sensations, feelings and emotions, what might they tell you?
- What is it they might need right now?
- How old do you feel when you're in touch with this place? Do you feel like the adult you or a younger part of you?
- Could the adult part of you attune to the younger part of you?

This resource allows those bodily sensations and impulses to resolve to a point of rest and stabilisation. And in that, we find regulation. It's also how we can make those ongoing, unintegrated and implicit memories a part of our autobiographical, explicit memory system. They are part of an old chapter of our story, and they no longer stop us from living fully in the present moment.

Often when we're stressed or ruminating about another person's behaviour we might find we're asking ourselves these sorts of questions:

- *Why do I think I feel this fear in relationships?*
- *Where did this fear come from?*
- *What did my family model in terms of relationships?*
- *What do I think is going to happen in my relationships when people don't respond to texts or when I don't know where they are?*

These may be interesting topics to explore and can certainly be useful when you're inside your window of tolerance, but they're more likely to keep you intellectualising what's happening rather than *feeling* what's happening in an embodied way – this may not be as helpful if you're dysregulated. This involves more thinking brain activity, and if we're overanalysing we may get stuck in our head, leading to more rumination, or obsessing over what another person is or isn't doing.

Tool 11: Examine your limiting beliefs and stories

Once you've looked into some areas of inaccurate thoughts, beliefs and stories, it can be helpful to take things one step further by gently interrogating your limiting beliefs and stories. One at a time, and only when you're feeling regulated, take each of your beliefs through the following exercise so you can find out where it came from, why it might have been useful at the time, and how it's continuing to impact you negatively today. Make a note of the belief and your answers in your notebook or journal, so that you can refer to them when you find yourself slipping into those negative thoughts.

1. Think of one of the beliefs you've identified and consider the following questions:
   - What did you say, to others and to yourself? How negative was your language?
   - Was what you said true?
   - Can you now say, with 100 per cent certainty, that your belief or prediction is true?

   This process will help you shift from automatically responding to certain situations and allow you to remap your nervous system. Even if you don't know whether a certain belief is true or not, questioning it is completely different from automatically assuming that you will fail or fall short, or that you're not good enough.
2. Consider what happens in your nervous system when you believe this. Maybe you notice resistance in your body. Perhaps there's a hollow ache of shame in your chest and belly and you want to give up on something. See if you can notice all the subtle changes you feel.
3. Ask yourself where this belief came from. If some of the feelings and emotions you identified in Step 2 feel familiar, you may already have an idea of how this belief came to be. If not, that's okay. See if you can recognise a previous challenging time where something similar occurred.

4. Now ask yourself how your brain is trying to protect you through this belief. Often we internalise these beliefs when our emotions are the strongest, to stop us from being hurt again, but consider these questions:
   - Does believing this really keep you safe?
   - What would your life be like if you were no longer living with this belief?

     Notice what happens in your body and what sensations you feel now.
   - What would you do differently if you were no longer living with this belief? Can you put this into action today?

Doing this will allow you to create agency and autonomy, which are both important for a healthy nervous system.

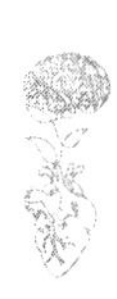

Because we know that chronic and traumatic stress can leave behind a neurological footprint, updating our internal roadmap, as you started to do in Chapter 7, is the key to learning to feel at home inside your body again. Interoception is a malleable system, and by using it, you can create lasting change. Improving interoceptive accuracy provides you with a compass and a clear, accurate map to get to where you want to go in life.

With a map updated to reflect your life as it is now, not how it was, you'll be equipped to navigate your way through life's twists and turns with inner resilience and a sense of openness and trust.

A stronger interoceptive system improves the hallmarks of good physiological balance, such as a robust immune response, healthy digestion and restful sleep.

When you redraw your old maps and also add new routes and references that include experiences of safety and connection, you can live in the present moment. You're not at the mercy of your outside environment, or at risk of being so easily overwhelmed. You give yourself the opportunity to explore life with a fresh curiosity and to make room for new stories.

10

Toolkit for shifting out of your too cold state

If you know you tend to spend long periods of time in your cold dorsal vagal state and dissociate from your bodily signals, it can be really helpful to set an alarm for three times a day to remind yourself to do a quick check-in with your bodily signals and get a reading on your nervous system thermostat.

Though several of the tools in this chapter are variations on the resources in the previous chapter for shifting out of the too hot state, some address the sense of disconnection or detachment many people feel in this colder dorsal vagal state. They often describe feeling removed from their surroundings or 'in a fog', alone in a cold dark room, and some may even dissociate or even feel they are floating away from their body. In these situations, containment resources such as the tapping exercise on page 276 and the light touch exercise on 281 can be excellent ways to find our way home to ourselves, and come back to our body.

The term 'containment' refers to the idea that the body is a container that holds everything we experience – emotions, thoughts, sensations, memories, and even our hopes and wishes. Containment resources work by helping us sense the actual physical container of our body and bringing our awareness back to the sensations of our body and skin. We're 'tapping in to' our exteroceptors here, with tactile information being sent to our brain.

Think of the way that tightly swaddling a crying baby can immediately calm them. A similar principle applies to dysregulated adults. Being reminded of our body by doing things such as tapping our skin gently or even hugging or holding ourselves can calm our nervous system. When we physically touch our body, we bring ourselves back into our body, back into the present.

Choosing tools for the cold state ❄

What do I feel tuning in to my nervous system?	What led me here?	What tools might help?
Helpless, collapsed. Strong urge to lie on the couch. Hopelessness. There's no use trying.	I opened the mail and there were several bills.	Gentle movement (page 274) Music playlist Putting my feet in the ocean
I notice shame. I feel like a fog has descended between me and the room. I feel alone, disconnected, like I'm wrong or bad.	I saw my friends at an event on Instagram and I wasn't invited.	Interoception Calling another friend Going to a park where there are people Asking why you weren't invited.

I feel hopeless and criticised. I can't take action. I feel activation inside me that makes me scared. I feel a sense of doom, as if something's about to go wrong.	My boss sent me an email that pointed out something I fell short on.	Creating a playlist to bring you out of your cold state (page 285) Crying

Bioplasticity tools

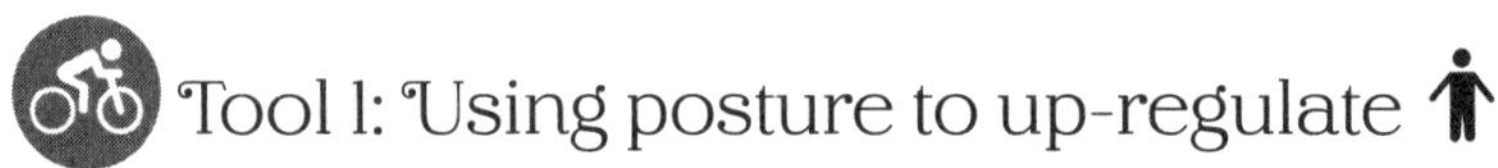

Tool 1: Using posture to up-regulate

In the previous chapter we used posture to help make our breathing more efficient when moving out of the sympathetic nervous system state, and we can do the same for the dorsal vagal state. In tandem with our breathing, we might move from lying down to an upright sitting position.

If we're feeling comfortable enough, and we find that sitting is helpful and brings us out of a state of hypoarousal, we might stand up. This will increase our blood pressure and provide more proprioceptive and interoceptive information to the brain, helping us return to our window of tolerance if we're in shutdown or freeze.

Movement-based tools

In this colder dorsal vagal state, we often feel collapsed and low in energy. This is the state where we can dissociate and become immobile. In Chapter 1, we met Samin, who went to a party reluctantly. She dreaded people asking about her relationship (which was over) or where she was living (she'd had to move back in with her parents). Samin felt ashamed of her circumstances and unwilling to be seen, and this was evident in the way she held her body and the low energy she brought to her interactions with other people. While sitting on the couch, she was slumped, her shoulders collapsed and hunched.

Reflect back on a time when you maybe had low energy and ruminating thoughts of shame like Samin. Once you tap in to that scenario, think about the sorts of resources your body might be craving, or the things you'd like to engage in that bring some energy into your body. Take out your notebook or journal and list five of these, near your window of tolerance map.

For Samin, engaging in light movement could have been an easy and effective way to introduce some sympathetic activation to her system, and bring her back to that ventral vagal just-right state where she could be comfortable and social. Before the party, a walk around the block or a light activity such as gardening could have given her energy and connected her to the present moment by orienting to her environment through her exteroceptors. Even at the party, simple things like standing up and walking around, or doing some micromovements such as wiggling her fingers and toes, might have been enough to nudge her back towards regulation.

Dorsal vagal: Gentle movements to energise	
Low energy	**High energy**
Imagining movement	Going to a park
Sitting on a therapy or fit ball	Moving limbs while lying
Tapping	Sit to stand
Walking	Marching

Tool 2: Tapping resource

We're going to utilise the tapping method, which is a containment resource. As a reminder, containment resources such as tapping help us connect with the sensory information of our body, which is especially helpful to turn up the 'volume' to the brain when we dissociate. This can be enough to keep important areas of the thinking brain online when we move into this state and we use our body to anchor us back to the present moment and return to regulation. You'll notice we integrate both the body-up (sensory) and brain-down (words).

1. Make a very relaxed fist with one hand while keeping your wrist relaxed as well. Then start gently tapping the inside of one arm, either in one place or moving up and down the arm slowly and gently. You might turn your arm over and begin tapping on the outside of your arm too. You can make the movements slower and rhythmic or faster and lighter. Experiment to see what suits your nervous system the best.
2. To help with the connection between your brain and your

body, keep your attention on the physical sensations in your body. Do they get louder with tapping? Next, notice what happens when you have the quiet thought, *This is my arm*. You're integrating both body-up and brain-down signals to shift you towards regulation.

3. Now make your way up your arm, onto your shoulder and across your chest. Again, mentally name each body part as you touch it, and notice what happens as you 'turn up the volume' on this sensory information.
4. If you're sitting down, you can stand up and practise tapping down the outside of your legs. You could try one at a time or do both together. Experiment with the amount of pressure and the speed. Over the bigger muscles you may find you'd like to try a firmer pressure. This can increase the sensory input to the brain, shifting you towards regulation.
5. Pay attention to the sensation of your knuckles tapping on your skin – the skin of your finger making contact with the skin of your arms and legs.
6. Bring your attention to your shift in energy and how your emotions might be changing as you use this resource. Record your answers to the following questions in your notebook or journal, under the heading 'Containment resource', close to your window of tolerance diagram.
   - Do you feel more anchored in your body?
   - Do you feel both physically and mentally light?
   - Do you feel more hopeful or more optimistic?
   - Do your thoughts feel quiet?

Eventually, as you move through this exercise, you should be able to bring yourself back to equilibrium. Of course, if you're in need of additional resources, or find that the tapping method isn't quite right for you, feel free to use some of the other resources we cover throughout this chapter, or any others listed in the table on pages 273–4.

When Tom, whom we met in Chapter 1, was struggling to spend time with his friends or focus on work after his mother died, a containment resource would have been an excellent tool. Tapping his arms, legs or forehead when he felt disconnected could help him move from shame-based thinking back into his body – and help re-establish that connection with his body.

Breathing tool

Breathing resources are common, but they aren't always the solution

Remember, if you're in a freeze or dissociated state, or a state of panic, paying attention to the breath can make you feel more dysregulated. If this is the case for you, try some of the other tools in this chapter instead. It's important to learn how to recognise what nervous system state you're in and how it changes as you try to use breathing resources. It's equally important to stop the moment you sense you might be triggered.

Tool 3: 2:1 breathing

In this state, our energy is conserved or even immobilised as a protective response. When this happens, our heart rate and blood pressure decrease, and our breaths per minute start to slow. In cases of an extreme shutdown, such as those Selena experienced in Chapter 5, someone might even experience bradycardia (when the heart slows to a dangerous level). This condition can cause us to feel dissociated, and even faint.

In order to exit this state and re-enter our window of tolerance, we can use a variation of the 1:2 breathing exercise included in the toolkit for the too hot state. Here, we'll also begin the exercise with 1:1 breathing and move into 2:1.

1. Find a position in which you can be both alert and relaxed. Often the dorsal vagal state brings a sense of collapse in the spine, but it's important to have some length through your spine to breathe effectively. Can you find a way to sit tall? The lungs don't have any skeletal muscles themselves, instead relying on the muscles of the ribcage, and we want to create the correct length-to-tension relationship so that your body can breathe efficiently.
2. Start by noticing your breath wherever it's easiest to feel. You might count the length of your in-breath first of all. How many counts does it take for you to breathe in? Next, count the length of your out-breath. How many counts does it take for you to breathe out?
3. Maintaining a sense of length through your spine, can you allow your breath to naturally deepen to a rhythm that's easy and natural?
4. Now shift towards a 1:1 breathing pattern by lengthening

by just one count whichever part of your breath was shorter. Keep a sense of length through your spine, and if you need to upregulate your system or you feel a sense of dissociation you might gently press your feet into the floor.

5. At this point you could try lengthening your in-breath by one count to add some sympathetic energy to your system. When we've disappeared into dorsal vagal collapse, breathing can help us mobilise energy in our nervous system.
6. What do you notice happens to your brain and body?
7. Now you could try lengthening your in-breath a little more and shortening your out-breath slightly. This can allow even more of the mobilising energy into our system. Remember to re-relax in your body when you do this, so you're not adding tension, especially your neck, shoulders and diaphragm.

Another body-up technique to use in combo with 2:1 breathing

If you feel disconnected from your body, try reconnecting before you continue.

1. Connect to the sensation of your feet on the floor by pressing them down into the ground. What do you notice?
2. Now rub your legs. In the cold dorsal vagal state, blood circulation moves away from the limbs towards the centre of the body. Rubbing your legs can help shift the blood flow back towards your legs. What do you notice?

Has 2:1 breathing helped to regulate you?

- Does your heart rate feel faster, similar to your normal set point?
- Does your breathing feel bigger, and more vibrant?
- What kinds of thoughts or stories are circulating in your brain, if any?

This type of resource would have been useful for Selena as it would have sped up her heart rate a bit, upregulating her just enough to feel less dissociated and flat. This would have helped move up her set point, and take her back towards her window of tolerance, and back to a state of feeling calm, more engaged in life and sociable.

Tool 4: Light touch for shifting out of the freeze state

In the extreme dorsal vagal state, we can experience freeze. In this state, the breath, not just the body, can become frozen. The muscles between our ribs (the intercostal) become tight and frozen.

In doing this exercise, you can come back into your body and out of the state of the freeze of dissociation. Of course, any of these resources, postures or breathing tools can be mixed and matched depending on your unique nervous system and your unique situation. You might just use posture, just use breathing, or use a combination of the two. Part of the embodied learning process is to work out what works well for you and learn to build a one-of-a-kind partnership with your heart–brain axis.

1. Place a hand on your chest, making contact with your skin. Imagine making contact with the muscles in your

chest, and try to feel the environment within as you breathe naturally.

2. As you breathe in, can you notice how your ribs lift slightly?
3. As you breathe out, can you feel how the ribs at the front of your chest lower slightly?
4. Can you move your spine with this naturally occurring pattern? The movements can be very small to start with and in time you can exaggerate them. As you make your movements larger, can your breath follow this movement so you naturally breathe deeper?

Posture tools

We can use posture to help make our breathing resources more efficient in moving out of the dorsal vagal state. In tandem with our breathing resources, we might, for example, move from lying down to an upright sitting position.

If we're feeling comfortable enough, and we find that sitting is helpful and brings us out of a state of hypoarousal, we might stand up. This increases our blood pressure and our heart rate, helping us return to our window of tolerance.

Tool 5: Using posture to shift out of your cold state

The following bioplasticity tool integrates exteroception, proprioception and the vestibular system. Every time you use it, you'll be training those systems and strengthening your vagal tone.

1. Sit in a chair in a way that allows you to be comfortable and alert. It's best if you're sitting in a chair with a full back

and no arms. You can close your eyes or simply look down to the floor and soften your gaze to bring your attention to your body.

2. Take a mental snapshot of your nervous system right now. Can you tell where your nervous system set point is at?
3. Begin by noticing your hands on your lap or resting on top of each other.
   - You might notice the warmth of your skin from one hand to the other.
   - Perhaps you can feel the material from your clothing on your hands.

   If it's hard to connect to your sensations because you feel dissociated from your body, rub your hands together a few times to increase the input to your brain from your body. If you find you're drifting away from the connection you may have had with your body, you could press one hand into the other, meeting the resistance. Experiment with how much pressure helps you to connect to your body.
4. To upregulate your nervous system, move from sitting to standing. Notice your feet connecting to the floor and the sensory information on the soles of your feet. You might notice the material on your floor (carpet, a rug or floorboards) or perhaps a sock or a shoe.
5. If you find it hard to connect to your body, notice what happens when you rub one foot back and forth on the floor several times and then reconnect to your sense of touch. Try it on both sides.
6. Press your feet into the floor so that the muscles in your

legs contract. See if you can keep your attention on the sensory information you receive.

7. To engage your vestibular system, rock your weight from your left to your right foot, keeping your attention on the soles of your feet. Can you find a rhythm that helps you connect to your body and upregulate your nervous system?
8. Finally, allow one foot to lift as you rock so that you spend some time balancing on one leg (you can hold onto a wall or bench if you need to).
9. How does it change your interoceptive accuracy? Is it easier to connect with sensations?

Did this posture exercise bring you back to regulation?

When you feel ready, return to stillness and take another mental snapshot of your brain–body system. Has it changed from earlier?

- What does your body feel like?
- Do you feel more 'in' your body?
- What sensations do you notice?
- What is your breath like?
- What urges or impulses come to mind?
- What thoughts do you notice?
- Do you feel more present 'in' your mind?
- How was your nervous system thermostat changed?

In your notebook or journal, write down anything you've noticed under the heading 'Postural regulation' near your window of tolerance map.

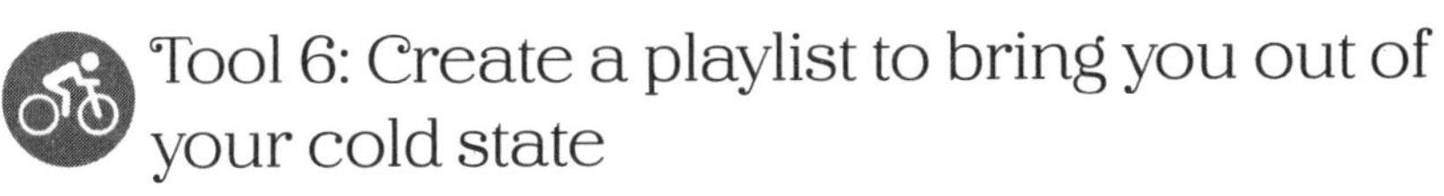

Tool 6: Create a playlist to bring you out of your cold state

When we find ourselves stuck in this colder dorsal vagal state – perhaps feeling sad or even filled with shame, music can be such an easy way to up-regulate ourselves. Which upbeat songs do you love? Which ones make you feel like dancing or remind you of happy memories and people you have fun with?

Take out your notebook or journal and list five songs that get your happy juices flowing. Now grab your phone and create a playlist. Give it a fun name and listen to it whenever you need a pick-me-up. Any time you discover a new song that fits this brief, add it to the playlist. If you notice that your posture starts to change while you listen to this music, lean in to those changes. If you feel like standing up, walking around or moving in any way while listening to this playlist, do that. The more systems you can engage in this upregulating process, the faster your brain will get the message that you're in a good place and ready to feel regulated again.

Tool 7: Create a playlist for finding your stillness state

Sometimes it's appropriate and even healthy for us to sit with sad, difficult feelings such as those we often associate with this dorsal vagal state. We don't want to get stuck here, of course, but giving ourselves time to feel a certain way and process hard emotions is essential if we want to return to true regulation afterwards.

Let's say you've just gone through a tough breakup. Before you can feel happy and light again, you'll likely need to 'feel all the feelings' and come to terms with no longer being part of a couple. You want to sit with any sadness without falling so far into it that you can't pull yourself out. To do this, you might create a playlist of songs about breakups so you can process the emotions you're feeling before moving on. Write a list in your notebook or journal songs that can support you as you process whatever tough emotions you're facing, then take out your phone and make a playlist.

Simple tools for co-regulation quick wins

Being stuck in a cold, immobile state where you're overwhelmed with tough emotions feels a lot like being in a cold room all by yourself. In times like this, it's so essential to lean in to co-regulation rather than listen to what our thinking brain's narrative is telling us to do when we're in dorsal vagal collapse – which might be to numb ourselves with TV or alcohol, comfort ourselves with food and withdraw from the world and from others even more. Those things might soothe us for an hour or two, but it won't be long before they trigger sensations that create more of those uncomfortable emotions, ultimately sinking us deeper into a blue, immobile state. You could try calling a friend or visiting the park.

If you're already deep in this state, you may not even feel able to talk to people. If so, can you find ways to communicate in baby steps? Could you text a friend? Or send them a voice message so you can hear their voice back without necessarily having a conversation? If you think of other ways to slowly bring yourself into communication with the outside world, make a note of them in your notebook or journal, so you can refer to them if you find yourself in this state again.

If you're up to it, try some of the activities below to get your social engagement system going. Make a list of your own ideas in your notebook or journal and add it to whenever you think of another.

Alone (with strangers or animals)	Together (with people you know)
Lie down with a pet and slowly stroke their fur, noticing the tactile information. Go the library and read around others (no need to talk). Volunteer to walk dogs at an animal shelter.	Take yourself to a public place where people are – like a park or a beach. Notice how you're not alone. Meet a family member for a coffee. Text a friend.

Now bring in brain-down regulation

We've explored some powerful body-up tools, but let's introduce some brain-down regulation to bring everything together. For a successful nervous system reset and future equilibrium, it's essential to integrate both body-up and brain-down information.

We know that the brain is a prediction machine and that because of this our perceptions are sometimes wrong. This may lead us to form mistaken (and often inflexible) beliefs. This also goes the other way – believing is seeing – that is, our perceptions are shaped by our brain-down expectations and assumptions about what we see, hear, and so on. When our prior expectations are mistaken, they powerfully influence us to perceive things in mistaken ways.

And so, once you're back in a comfortable, secure and regulated state, take a look at the areas of your life where limiting beliefs and old narratives could be influencing you. You may notice when you move into the dorsal vagal state there are familiar stories or thoughts: *I'm unlovable, It never works out for me, I'll always be alone* or *There's something wrong with me.* Finding those predictions and stories will allow you to uncouple them mentally from the sensory information you receive from moment to moment.

You might recall how Lisa, whom we met in the Introduction could identify and experience the fear, but she still had unresolved reactions. Once she could identify and experience these reactions physically (body-up processing), they gradually loosened their grip on her. With practice, she learned to identify and observe the bodily signals and impulses in her body from when she was a child, and to use tools and physical actions that interrupted those maladaptive responses.

Just as communication between the body and brain is bidirectional, so is the feedback between the survival brain and the thinking brain. As we become more aware of the sensations and impulses of the body when stress arousal is high, and learn to process them, we will experience a positive influence on our emotions and thinking, and vice versa. If, on the other hand, we use brain-down strategies to manage what's happening in our body, we may intellectualise, ignore, suppress or fail to support adaptive body processes, and fail to resolve dysregulation from past trauma.

This following exercise is one of the most valuable things you can do to help reset your nervous system.

Tool 8: Locate your areas of faulty neuroception

Sarah had recently started sharing her pottery creations on Instagram, hoping one day to make some money from it. Her followers were almost always positive, but after growing her audience she became more and more nervous about sharing her products.

One day, after putting up a new vase she'd spent hours on, a comment appeared that dropped Sarah into her dorsal vagal state. 'This is so expensive! You're taking advantage of people so you can live a privileged life.' Sarah was devastated, she certainly hadn't had a privileged upbringing, in fact, her parents had worked so much that she often spent time in after-school care. Sarah felt the familiar hollow ache of shame engulfing her. Then a second comment came through: 'This woman is so annoying'.

Sarah felt herself collapse, and felt an impending sense of doom. She left the pottery studio, went home and fell onto her bed. For hours she lay there, feeling completely alone and abandoned. A memory came to mind of when she was a pre-teen and at a friend's birthday party. When she went to the bathroom all the girls had left the room and there was a note 'Sarah is so annoying'. It had devastated Sarah and she recognised that familiar sense of not belonging. Soon after, Sarah's partner came home and held her on the bed as she cried. Sarah said she was giving up pottery and closing down her Instagram account. They stayed there for over an hour.

It took some time but she felt herself move out of collapse and her partner encouraged her not to give up. Sarah had been using some resources to up-regulate her out of her dorsal vagal state that helped shift her out of a shame spiral. She learned to recognise and attune to the bodily signals that flagged that she was heading towards the cold state and she realised that this was her default when she felt herself move out of her comfort zone. Sarah had other memories arise in the following weeks related to her alcoholic mother which she grieved and processed, and she eventually joined the dots between this and her current default responses to criticism. With her partner's support she blocked the people who'd made those nasty comments and continued on with making and sharing her pottery.

Again, this is where we can use interoception to help cultivate regulation and attune to physical sensations and impulses as they move through our body, and sift through the thoughts that arise. Try sitting in a way where you can be as comfortable as possible, let your attention shift to your body, and slowly allow your attention to shift to where you feel shame, hopelessness or helplessness. You might mentally whisper what sensations are arising and allow them to be just as they are. If you feel dissociated or disconnected, you might like to try this standing up or gently press your feet into the floor while seated. You can ask the following questions:

- How does this shame, hopelessness or helplessness show up in your body?
- How does it feel to be 'in touch' with what's here?
- If you could pass a microphone to these sensations, feelings and emotions, what might they tell you?
- What is it they might need right now?
- How old do you feel when you're in touch with this place? Do you feel like the adult you or a younger part of you?
- Could the adult part of you attune to the younger part of you?

- Does this sensory experience feel familiar to something from your past?

This resource allows those bodily sensations and impulses to resolve to a point of rest and stabilisation. And in that, we find regulation. It's also how we can make those ongoing, unintegrated implicit memories a part of our autobiographical, explicit memory system. They are part of an old chapter of our story and stop living in the present moment.

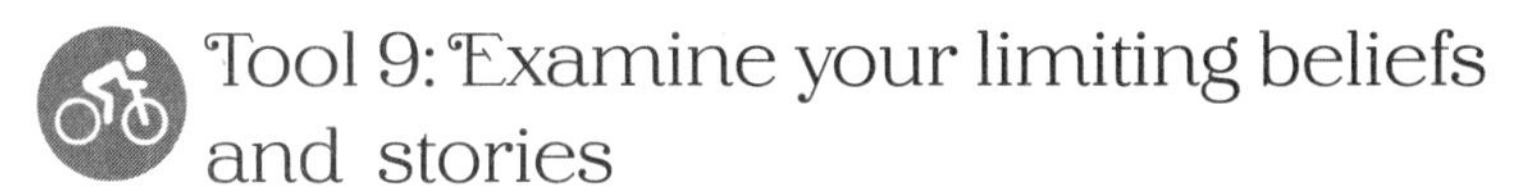

Tool 9: Examine your limiting beliefs and stories

By now you will have identified some areas of limited beliefs or unhelpful narratives that, like Sarah, may be stopping you from doing what it is you'd truly love to be doing. From here, you might want to take things a step further by gently interrogating limiting beliefs and stories. To do this, turn to page 268 and complete Tool 11 in the previous chapter. It applies equally here.

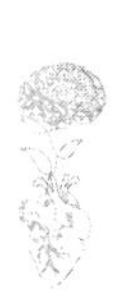

You're now equipped with lots of tools for returning to your window of tolerance from either a too hot or too cold state and ultimately resetting your nervous system. In the next chapter you'll learn some lifestyle tools that will help you consolidate those gains and maintain equilibrium well into the future.

11

Lifestyle tools to support your reset

To solidify all you've learned about your nervous system and build confidence in your body's ability to support you the way it was designed to, we're going to explore a few practical lifestyle tools. Implementing changes in any (or all) of these key areas will add to your physical health, as well as that of your brain–body system, by creating optimal conditions for a nervous system reset to occur.

Your lifestyle may already include many of the suggestions in this chapter. If so, you're starting from a good spot. If not, there are so many small tweaks you can make today. There's no need to dramatically overhaul your routine or diet overnight, either. In the same way the tiniest gut microbe influences our wellness, the smallest, incremental changes can influence our health and support our nervous system in quite profound ways.

The first area we'll look at probably won't come as a surprise, since you already know the importance of the gut–brain axis, and specifically the microbiota, in regulating the nervous system.

What may surprise you, however, is how large an influence external factors have over the health of our gut microbiota, and how easy it can be to boost microbiota health by using those to our advantage.

As babies, the way we are born (vaginal birth versus caesarean section) and the way we are fed (breast milk versus formula) have a big influence on the health and diversity of our microbiota. And from our first day out of the womb, the influences just keep coming! The environment we live in, the people (and animals) we share space with and the things we touch all contribute to the unique fingerprint that is our microbiota. The microorganisms of the microbiota colonise many parts of the human body, including the skin, but those in the gut are very important when it comes to the nervous system.

By adulthood, the average gut microbiota is fairly stable, but this can change drastically, when we endure long periods of illness or stress, or need to take antibiotics – since those kill gut bacteria indiscriminately – good or bad. It can also change drastically depending on our diet. The gut tells our nervous system when we're dysregulated, and our brain responds accordingly.

Although it's nothing to do with the gut microbiota, this gut–brain connection is one reason why low blood sugar levels can make us feel dizzy, lightheaded or even dissociated (which we might associate with the colder dorsal state). Alternatively, eating or drinking things that spike blood sugar can nudge us towards the sympathetic nervous system state, and make us feel jittery, anxious or on edge. It makes sense that if we eat less of the foods that cause these extreme effects, and fuel ourselves with foods that regulate us or bring us back to homeostasis, our brain will regulate in kind. Since what we put into our bodies is one of the external factors we have the most control over, let's start there.

The many benefits of the Mediterranean diet

The Mediterranean diet gets its name from the eating patterns found in the countries around the Mediterranean Sea. It's not so much a 'diet' as a lifestyle that embraces plenty of fresh food, nuts, legumes and seafood, and far less red meat and sugar than the typical 'Western' diet. Like the people who've thrived on this way of eating for thousands of years, you can follow the parts you like and discard those you don't.

The Mediterranean diet

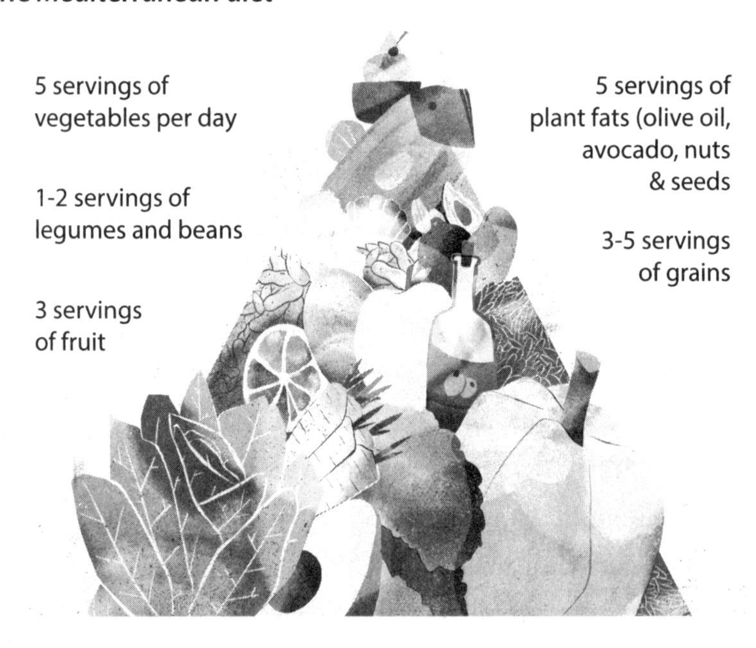

Fibre-rich diets like this one support brain function, promote heart health and regulate blood sugar levels, all of which contribute to how regulated (or not) we are. Additionally, the Mediterranean diet boasts an anti-inflammatory effect thanks to polyphenols – a group of plant micronutrients with prebiotic (i.e. microbiota-feeding) and antioxidant properties.

Olive oil – a central ingredient in most Mediterranean dishes – has high levels of these polyphenols, along with protective antioxidants. Polyphenols are also found in colourful fruits and vegies, herbs, spices, dark chocolate, tea and coffee. These ingredients can be considered 'good mood foods' since they've also been associated in some studies with a lower risk of depression. Any time you add more colour to your plate by eating a variety of plant foods, you're boosting your polyphenols and that gut microbiome diversity.

While there's no blueprint for the perfect healthy microbiota, research tells us that a healthy gut is one that has a wide diversity of gut bacteria. Diverse microbiotas are considered more resilient because they support the immune system and can help to fight off potential infections. When it comes to creating a diverse and resilient microbiome, the principles of the Mediterranean diet apply: eat a range of vegetables, fruits, legumes and wholegrains.

On the other hand, a Western diet that's low in plant foods but high in ultra-processed, fried and sugar-rich foods is associated with a less diverse microbiome. Given the relationship between the gut and our overall physical and mental wellbeing, lower gut diversity has been associated in some studies with various health conditions, including obesity, asthma and allergies, and some mental illnesses. Associations have also been observed in some studies between a diet high in processed foods and increased occurrence of depression and anxiety. Processed foods increase inflammation, which is increasingly being implicated as one possible cause of depression and also fatigue.

In the landmark SMILEs trial, researchers at the Food and Mood Centre at Deakin University found that a 12-week Mediterranean-style dietary intervention was significantly associated with improved depressive symptoms. This finding has been replicated in several other trials since.

Probiotics and prebiotics

Fermented dairy and fresh produce contain probiotics and prebiotics, respectively, and both are hugely important for gut health. Please note, the following information is not intended as a substitute for professional advice given by your healthcare or medical professional.

Probiotics

Probiotics are live bacteria that can be consumed to provide physical and mental health benefits. They're found naturally in fermented foods such as yoghurt, kefir, miso or sauerkraut, and can also be taken as supplements. Fermented foods or probiotic supplements are an easy way of adding more 'good' bacteria to the gut, increasing its diversity and leaving less room for 'bad' bacteria to flourish. In turn, this enables the entire gut microbiome to produce beneficial compounds for the rest of the body to use.

Numerous studies have associated taking probiotics with a range of health benefits, from significantly reducing depression and anxiety symptoms in postpartum women, to alleviating anxiety symptoms in chronic fatigue patients and improving cortisol regulation, immune system function and sleep quality in IBS sufferers.

This is as easy as adding a heaped tablespoon of brine-fermented pickles or sauerkraut to your plate or eating natural yoghurt each day.

If that's too much of a stretch, you can find probiotic supplements in the health aisles of almost every supermarket or pharmacy.

Yoghurt

One of the best sources of probiotics, yoghurt is milk fermented by probiotics, especially lactic acid bacteria and bifidobacteria. Choose yoghurt with active or live cultures and avoid those with high amounts of added sugar even if it's labelled low-fat or fat-free. Some yoghurts are marketed as probiotic, but any unflavoured, pot-set natural yoghurt will contain probiotics.

Sauerkraut

Traditional sauerkraut is finely shredded cabbage that has been fermented in brine by lactic acid bacteria. You can use it as a side dish with meat and once it is made it can be stored in an airtight container for months. It's a traditional food popular in many countries, especially Eastern Europe. Other fermented vegetables are also commonly sold as 'krauts'.

In addition to its probiotic qualities, sauerkraut is rich in fibre, which makes it a prebiotic as well.

Tempeh

This fermented soybean product is a common meat substitute. Its flavour is nutty or similar to that of mushrooms, and it's an excellent addition to stir-fries. Double points if you include lots of fibre-rich prebiotic vegetables.

Prebiotics

Prebiotics are foods that contain indigestible fibre. While our own digestive tract cannot break this fibre down, our 'good' bacteria use it as food, which improves the balance of our microbiota.

Increasing our intake of prebiotics is a very simple way to boost nervous system health. The list of prebiotic foods (see below) is extensive, and includes many vegetables, fruits, legumes, grains and nuts. A well-rounded, balanced diet that includes plenty of these foods will ensure that your 'good' bacteria are well fed. This enhances immunity, helps the body absorb essential minerals and allows our 'good' bacteria to produce anti-inflammatory compounds.

While upping the fresh produce you eat will ensure you're getting plenty of prebiotics, the ingredients listed below are examples of foods that are particularly rich in prebiotics.

Vegetables	Fruit	Legumes	Grains	Nuts
Artichokes	Apples	Chickpeas	Rye	Cashews
Asparagus	Berries	Kidney beans	Wheat	Almonds
Jerusalem artichokes	Pears	Lentils	Barley	Hazelnuts
Onion	Persimmons			
Garlic	Watermelon			
Leeks				
Mushrooms				

Movement and exercise

We've explored some of the ways that movement is important for neuroplasticity and as a resource for regulating the nervous system, but regular exercise can also have a similar and ongoing positive impact on our brain–body system, regardless of our nervous system state. Exercise positively influences the entire body, from the heart, lungs, gut and fascia to mental health.

When it comes to treating depression, a recent study showed that physical activity was one and a half times more effective than counselling or the leading medications. That's not to say that counselling and medication should be replaced with exercise, but it suggests that exercise could be widely adopted as a first-choice treatment.

When we talk about exercising more, that doesn't have to mean hitting the gym for intense cardio or weight training sessions (though these can be great for us). Simple, moderate-intensity exercise – aka movement – done regularly is beneficial to us in *so* many ways. Regular movement:

- improves the normal functioning of the immune system
- has a positive influence on the endocrine system, for example, by stimulating the production of human growth hormone (HGH), which helps maintain normal body structure and metabolism
- promotes better sleep (which is when the body releases the most HGH)
- helps control blood sugar levels, metabolism and blood pressure
- enhances cardiac function by increasing heart rate,

constricting blood vessels and increasing blood pressure, which helps to distribute blood to active tissues, carrying the energy and oxygen they need
- reduces adrenaline levels at rest, leading to a reduction in the stressed feelings that adrenaline causes
- increases dopamine levels in the brain, decreasing stress, depression and that uneasy feeling created by stress
- increases serotonin levels, which can positively impact mood, appetite, digestion, memory and sleep
- reduces inflammation
- improves body composition
- positively influences gut microbiota.

Ideally, adults should get 150 minutes of moderate-intensity physical activity per week. This might be made up of things like:

- cycling 8 kilometres (5 miles) in 30 minutes
- swimming laps for 20 minutes
- doing water aerobics for 30 minutes
- walking 3 kilometres (2 miles) in 30 minutes
- playing a match of doubles tennis
- pushing a lawn mower for 30 minutes
- dancing for 30 minutes.

The key to improving your health is identifying a sustainable exercise or form of movement that can become part of your everyday routine. This means it has to be something you *enjoy* doing, that you have time to do, that you can afford to do and that is accessible to you (e.g. there's no point choosing reformer Pilates if there's no studio near you).

Exercise and pain

Unfortunately, many people experience pain all the time. Central sensitisation is a condition of the central nervous system (brain and spinal cord) that is associated with the development and maintenance of persistent pain. When central sensitisation occurs, the nervous system goes through a process called *wind-up* and gets regulated in a persistent state of high reactivity. This state lowers the threshold for what causes pain, which means that pain persists even after the initial injury might have healed.

As a physiotherapist, I saw firsthand how debilitating persistent pain can be, and the impact it can have on a person's lifestyle, so if you've given up activities you love to avoid pain, I empathise. Often, friends and family tell us to 'listen to our body' or 'let pain be our guide', but this isn't always helpful, because it can cause you swing between the highs and lows of an 'overdo/underdo' cycle where you exercise in the absence of pain and stop moving when it returns. This cycle closely resembles the swinging that can occur with dysregulation – between the highs of anxiety and the lows of shutdown.

When we pull back on movement to avoid pain, we might feel better in the short term, but in the longer term less movement leads to declining fitness levels and eventually to less social interaction, because reduced mobility and fitness makes moving around in the world so much more challenging.

Others might take a totally different approach to pain by trying to ignore it. They push harder, determined not to let pain beat them. Frustratingly, though, more pain lies at the end of both of these roads. Pushing harder often leads to pain flares, and avoiding activity completely leads to more pain and disability.

Activity pacing

If a condition such as fibromyalgia, persistent pain, chronic fatigue syndrome or frequently collapsing into dorsal vagal shutdown is keeping you from getting your 150 minutes of exercise a week, 'activity pacing' can be a really effective tool to get you heading in the right direction. Activity pacing is exactly what it sounds like: it's when we pace an activity around your specific needs and abilities so you can work steadily towards a long-term goal. Pacing is important in pain management, because it helps you to stay active, maintain physical fitness and strength, and keep doing the things you care about or need to do, while also helping you avoid pain flares (or crash into the dorsal vagal state).

Using this approach to movement can be great for helping you find the middle ground between overexercising and underexercising. Think of it like that diagram on page 30 – ideally, you want to be working within a 'window of tolerance', but also gradually increasing the amount of activity you do (i.e. loading the system) over time. This way, you're in that upper level of that window, in the 'stretch zone', where your fitness and abilities can improve.

When using a paced approach to deal with pain, it's best to focus on doing activities that can be measured in some way – either in duration, distance or number of repetitions. This way, you have a clear target and limit, and this gives you a basis from which to build activity tolerance, which is important to allow you to do everyday tasks. Your paced activity might be walking around the local area for 10 minutes, or vacuuming the house for 15 minutes.

You've probably heard the phrase 'Use it or lose it'. Well, after years of helping patients with persistent pain, one of my favourite sayings is 'Motion is lotion'. I encourage you to use a pacing journal (see below), whether you suffer from persistent pain or chronic fatigue syndrome, or you're new to exercise or trying to get back into it after a long time.

Exercise: Activity pacing for pain, chronic fatigue and Long Covid

Before beginning this process, it's important to know the difference between a pain flare and regular muscle soreness. It's normal for pain to increase *after* an activity – especially if that activity engaged muscles you haven't used in a while. If you have chronic shoulder pain, for example, you may be able to wash your windows comfortably for 30 minutes. Your shoulder may feel a bit achy afterwards but return to its normal baseline by the following day. If, however, you wash windows for 40 minutes, and feel achy afterwards, and the pain gets progressively worse and is bad the next day, that's a pain flare, and it's your body's way of telling you that you've done too much.

1. Write a list of activities you *need* to do and *want* to do. It's good to pick regularly from both rather than just the things that need to get done.
2. Choose an activity you can measure and then go and do it. If yours is walking, estimate how long you could walk for without getting a flare up or exhausted. Then, go for a walk and measure how long or far you go.
3. Write this number down and if the following day you're not exhausted and you don't have a flare-up of symptoms, set this as your baseline. For example, if you experienced a little pain but could continue fairly comfortably for 30 minutes and the

next day you were a little achy but could still carry on, that's your baseline.

4. Take three measures over three days to get an average (by adding the three results together, then dividing that by three). If you like, you could reduce this number by 10 per cent to give yourself a buffer to account for other activities you may be doing during the day. The number you arrive at is your baseline for Week 1. Write this down in your notebook or journal, or in a specific pacing journal.
5. Do this activity daily for a week with the goal of meeting your Week 1 baseline number. After each day, evaluate how you're feeling using a notebook or journal, and if you feel able to, increase the time, distance or number of repetitions by 10 per cent. The number you are comfortably able to achieve by the end of the week becomes your baseline for Week 2, and so on.

Don't overdo it!

It's important to take regular, scheduled rests and relaxation breaks, even on the days you're feeling good, because those are the days where it's easy to overdo it. Adding short rests before and after particularly stressful or demanding tasks is also important. Practising relaxation, stretching and daily walks, even on your not-so-good days, will also help to control the pain. Slowly but surely, you're conditioning your body for activity and training it to do that activity for longer and more comfortably each day – yet another example of bioplasticity in action.

Animals

There is a lot of research to support the regulating effect animals have on us. If you don't have enough people for co-regulation, volunteering at an animal shelter can provide animal co-regulation, and you'll be around like minded people as well. Or you might take the time to pat a friendly dog or cat while running errands, or play with a friend's or family member's pet while visiting their house. Pets are good for us on several levels that aid nervous system regulation. From a co-regulation perspective, time spent with a much-loved pet can lower blood pressure and reduce stress.

On a microbial level, the bacteria we pick up from living with an animal contributes to that all-important gut diversity. Dogs in particular have been linked with a healthier gut and a more balanced microbiota and, in turn, a stronger immune system. Children who grow up with dogs tend to have a better balanced microbiota, depending on how early they were exposed to the dog.

Assistance dogs

These dogs are trained to support people following trauma. The benefits include:

- **Co-regulation:** Interacting with a therapy dog has been found to reduce symptoms of anxiety and depression, decrease physiological arousal (such as heart rate and blood pressure), and improve social skills. Animal-intervention programs in hospitals suggested various benefits, such as reducing stress, pain and anxiety.
- **Contact:** Physical contact with dogs facilitates tactile input to the body, which is important for shifting our

of dissociation and shutdown, and for co-regulation, grounding and focus. When we pat a dog or allow a dog to snuggle up on our lap or beside us, our body releases oxytocin, a hormone that helps reduce stress and anxiety. This shifts us towards our window of tolerance.

- **Nightmare interruption:** Assistance dogs are trained to recognise signs of distress in sleep or immediately after waking, and provide calming support.
- **Positioning cues:** An assistance dog can create space for its owner in public or crowded places, allowing for an increased sense of security and encouraging social engagement.

Equine therapy or hippotherapy

Hippotherapy means treatment with the aid of a horse from the Ancient Greek *hippos*, meaning 'horse', and *therapeia*, meaning 'attendance'. Riding a horse with assistance can improve motor control, postural control, coordination, balance, attention, sensory processes and performance in daily activities. This is a way to improve the communication of the brain–body system through:

- **the vestibular system:** balancing on the horse as it moves and changes direction
- **proprioception:** adjusting our posture on the horse and being aware of our own body
- **interoceptive accuracy:** movement that can help us interocept with greater accuracy
- **exteroception:** targetting our tactile, visual and auditory systems simultaneously

If you have the means of accessing hippotherapy or horse riding, it can be of enormous benefit. Often we need to be aware of our own state if we're working with horses – this is an excellent way to cultivate your own autonomic awareness.

Sleep

Sleep is absolutely vital for the healthy functioning of *all* our bodily systems. If we have poor sleep over many months or years, we make poor dietary choices, throw off our natural eating rhythm (i.e. the timing of our meals), and even destabilise the hormones that cue feelings of appetite and hunger. Most notably, perhaps, is the link between sleep and stress, and the way getting too little sleep causes us to feel more stressed.

Chronic sleep deprivation can result in lower HRV, which means the vagal brake isn't functioning properly. When this happens we know that allostasis is impacted, and so, for example, blood pressure can arise. Not surprisingly chronic sleep deprivation is linked with hypertension and has several ongoing dysregulating effects on the brain–body system. It impacts the ventral vagal state, which in turn impacts our social engagement system, emotional wellbeing, recovery functions and vagal brake.

Sleep deprivation also impacts our hormonal or endocrine system by affecting cortisol levels. Cortisol plays an important role in our circadian rhythm, peaking in the early morning and mobilising our energy for waking. We may produce more cortisol when sleep-deprived and this impacts our stress activation, metabolism and immune system. That stress in turn impacts our other systems as well as our microbiota.

Growing evidence also suggests that the gut microbiota can influence sleep quality. While short periods of too little sleep or interrupted sleep, won't have much of an impact on gut health, too little sleep over the long term can have a dramatic impact, since the link between sleep and the gut microbiota is bidirectional: poor sleep means worsening conditions for microbiota, and poor digestive health leads to issues with sleep.

Here are a few simple tips to prepare your nervous system for sleep:

- Limit your use of electronic devices in the hour before bed. It's good to limit other sources of blue light, such as TV, and you may also wish to dim the lights.
- See if you can get to bed and get up at roughly the same time each day. It's best if you're in bed before 11 pm.
- Try to spend time in natural daylight each day – even better if it's early in the morning, to help with your morning cortisol response.
- Try to make exercise a part of your regular routine, as it's known to improve sleep quality.
- Avoid caffeine after 2 pm, particularly if you're sensitive to caffeine.

Exercise: Falling to sleep

To fall asleep, we need to move into the blended state of stillness (the combination of the dorsal vagal cool state and the ventral vagal just-right state; see page 56). This means winding back the sympathetic nervous system – and that's not always easy to do if we've had a stressful day. Rather than lying there tossing and turning, get up and do some gently slow movement to discharge the stress activation.

1. Slowly circle your arms overhead and back down, breathing in as you raise them and exhaling as you lower them. Notice any signs of stress activation discharge, such as yawning, sighing or bodily relief. You may notice those looping thoughts finally stop.
2. Lie on your back with your knees bent: gently rock your knees to one side as you breathe in, then breath out as you return to centre. Repeat to the other side and continue for as long as feels beneficial.
3. Still lying on your back, straighten your legs and try to move to 1:2 breathing (see page 255) to encourage your nervous system to shift out of sympathetic activation. Aim to be closer to your window of tolerance before getting back into bed.

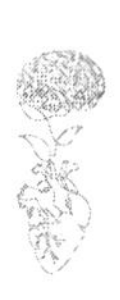

As you implement these lifestyle changes, make sure you go gently and gradually, so that you can sustain them in the long term. That will allow you greater success not only in resetting your nervous system, but also in keeping your set point exactly where it should be.

CONCLUSION
This isn't the end

I'm hoping that the frameworks and tools I've shared in this book have helped you tune in to your nervous system and hear what it's telling you. When we map the territory of our internal world and can understand what's happening in our remarkable brain–body system, we gain so much power and autonomy over our life and our health.

The roller-coaster experiences of life can often take us by surprise, and the sensations and feelings that come up as a result can often feel frightening. We might sometimes feel as if we're a helpless passenger along for the ride, but that's not the reality. If we can tether ourselves to a regulated state as we navigate our inner world, we can build confidence in our ability to handle situations, and in our inner resilience to come back to centre afterwards. Regardless of how overwhelmed or out of control life may feel for you today, it's more than possible to find your way back to a calmer, more balanced way of living.

The guideposts of your nervous system states are like unique landmarks in your roadmap. The more awareness you give to how you feel, think and behave in each state, the more visible your landmarks will become to you, and the easier it will be to recognise where you are, how you ended up there and the best route back home.

Your knowledge of how your internal and external senses feed into the predictions made by your brain can help you pinpoint *why* you're feeling a particular way. You'll be able to look more objectively at your emotions and question whether your responses are grounded in your current reality or in your brain's expectations about how things *might* unfold.

When we understand that none of our nervous states is inherently bad, and that each one of them exists to protect and serve us in some way, it's easier to embrace them for the benefits they provide us in certain moments. Flowing in and out of these states as change demands is a natural part of human existence. And while it's not normal to get stuck in one of these states for a long time, it's understandable that this happens, given the pace and challenges of modern life. Falling into dysregulation isn't your fault, and it's not something you should blame or scold yourself for.

Treating yourself with compassion and understanding goes a long way to bringing you back to centre. With the knowledge and resources in this book, you can consciously steer your system back to regulation, and repeat this process over and over again. When these processes become routine, noticing a shifting of state in the moment and taking steps to regulate that if necessary becomes as automatic as breathing.

At its core, nervous system regulation is about building our ability to regulate and support ourselves in the face of challenges, and then either adapting to or recovering from those challenges with a minimum of negative consequences for our wellbeing.

This is true resilience. To my mind, the mainstream definition of resilience seems to paint a picture of the glory of soldiering on, no matter what, during tough times. To me that's not resilience. Learning to do the best we can with the nervous system we have, and using regulation and resources to minimise the harm that stress and trauma can have on us – that's true resilience.

In this context, we accept that it's *okay* – even normal – to get stressed. It's also perfectly *okay to struggle* when facing hard things. I measure my own resilience by my ability to move through life's challenges and return to my centre, and in doing so I grow and evolve. This process gets messy, but as long as we give ourselves grace and permission to make mistakes, we can transform towards wholeness. As much as I've learned about my nervous system and as many tools as I've collected, there's always more to learn. Each phase of life comes with its own highs and lows. The pressures we face in our twenties won't be the same ones we tackle in our forties. The more life we live, the more necessary it becomes to remind ourselves that our past experiences don't accurately predict our future.

A regulated body–brain system is one that's able to respond to the situations we're actually in rather than the ones we predict we're about to be in. This, above all, is what makes it possible for us to enjoy life in a more balanced and comfortable way.

Acknowledgements

When I look back at the journey of where this all began it's been more than two-and-a-half years!

I was first approached by a small publishing house to see if I would be interested in writing a book. Whilst they weren't quite the right fit for me, a seed was planted.

Call it fate, but I was connected with the right people at the right time, and *The Nervous System Reset* was born shortly after my daughter, Ivy.

Writing this book in the final trimester of my pregnancy with swollen ankles and the relentless heat meant many trips to the swimming pool and an ongoing coaxing of my nervous system back towards regulation so I could complete my best work.

The unwavering co-regulation and support from my husband – who believed in the vision of this book well before I did – is one of the main reasons it exists today. Indra, thank you for your stability, care, cheerleading and wisdom. I love and appreciate you so much.

To the Nervous System School team who've supported me throughout the writing process, celebrated the exciting times and are creating events to share this work with the readers who need it – thank you!

To my agent, Anna Geller, thank you for understanding my vision for this book and how the world so needs it right now. I'm honoured to be your first Australian author and thank you for helping me navigate the publishing world.

Thank you to Ingrid Ohlsson, Rebecca Lay, Katie Bosher, Nicola Young and the Pan Macmillan Australia team for your help in editing and polishing the manuscript. I'd also like to thank the Balance and Bluebird teams who jumped at the chance to publish in the US and UK, and who have been so positive over the last two-and-a-half years.

Thank you to the talented illustrator, Jake Minton, for bringing so much fun to the process and the book! I've loved working with you.

Thank you to Dr Stephen Porges for your incredible research, which has helped thousands of clinicians and patients join the dots. I'm honoured to share this research.

Thank you Professor Lorimer Moseley for your teaching concepts on pain and the brain–body connection – and for getting my humour when I asked you if you were the Dr Phil of the physio world!

I'd also like to thank the countless teachers I've had over the years at Curtin University, the researchers I was fortunate enough to assist and learn from and, after graduating, those who taught me to see things with new eyes and made me richer for it. This includes Dr Toby Hall and Paula Raymond-Yacoub.

Thank you to my mentors Jack Kornfield and Tara Brach for inspiring me and igniting within me a deep commitment to my life's purpose.

Endnotes

6 Our brain is a 'prediction machine' and . . .: Lisa Fieldman Barrett et al., 'Interoceptive predictions in the brain', *Nature reviews. Neuroscience*, vol. 16, no. 7, 2015, pp. 419–29.

7 Regulation turns into dysregulation and . . .: Gail A. Alvares et al., 'Autonomic nervous system dysfunction in psychiatric disorders and the impact of psychotropic medications: a systematic review and meta-analysis', *Journal of Psychiatry and Neuroscience*, vol. 41, no. 2, 2026, pp. 89–104.

8 Provided we get to recover fully from stress . . .: Bruce S. McEwen, 'Allostasis and Allostatic Load: Implications for Neuropsychopharmacology', *Neuropsychopharmacology*, vol. 22, 2000, pp. 108–124

9 The same is true of traumatic stress . . .: Bruce S. McEwen, 'Allostasis and Allostatic Load: Implications for Neuropsychopharmacology', *Neuropsychopharmacology*, vol. 22, 2000, pp. 108–124; Jenny Guidi et al., 'Allostatic Load and Its Impact on Health: A Systematic Review', *Psychotherapy and psychosomatics*, vol. 90, no. 1, 2021, pp. 11–27.

9 Cortisol gets a bad rap for being . . .: Lauren Tahu et al., *Physiology, Cortisol*, StatPearls Publishing, Florida, 2024.

9 Prolonged periods of stress can cause fluctuations . . .: Bart G. Oosterholt et al., 'Burnout and cortisol: Evidence for a lower cortisol awakening response in both clinical and non-clinical burnout', Journal of Psychosomatic Research, vol. 78, no. 5, 2015.

10 This is because trauma is subjective and . . .: National Registry of Evidence-based Programs and Practices, 'Behind the term: trauma', *CalSWEC*, 2016, calswec.berkeley.edu

10 It leads to a fragmentation, a dissociation that . . .: Ono van der Hart et al., 'Trauma-related dissociation: conceptual clarity lost and found', *The Australian and New Zealand Journal of Psychiatry*, vol. 38, no. 11–12, 2004; Catherine Classen et al., 'Trauma and dissociation', *Bulletin of the Menninger Clinic*, vol. 57,

no. 2, 1993; Martin J. Dorahy et al., 'Relationship between trauma and dissociation: A historical analysis', in Eric Vermetten et al., *Traumatic dissociation: Neurobiology and treatment*, American Psychiatric Publishing, 2007.

11 The exact point at which we label or judge . . .: Peter Payne et al., 'Somatic experiencing: using interoception and proprioception as core elements of trauma therapy', *Frontiers in Psychology*, vol. 6, 2015.

11 This impacted her immune system, which caused . . .: François M. Abboud et al., 'Autonomic Neural Regulation of the Immune System: Implications for Hypertension and Cardiovascular Disease', *Hypertension*, vol. 59, no. 4, 2012, pp. 755–62.

14 Our bodies simply can't be talked out . . .: Stephen W. Porges, 'Polyvagal Theory: A Science of Safety', *Frontiers in Integrative Neuroscience*, vol. 16, 2022.

14 If you're just beginning to learn about . . .: Manos Tsakiris et al., 'Interoception beyond homeostasis: affect, cognition and mental health', *Philosophical Transactions of the Royal Society B*, vol. 371, no. 1780, 2016.

14 Those same thoughts, beliefs and emotions . . .: Donald D. Price, *Psychological Mechanisms of Pain and Analgesia*, IASP Press, Michigan, 1999; National Advisory Committee on Health and Disability and Accident Compensation Corporation, *Guide to Assessing Psychosocial Yellow Flags in Acute Low Back Pain: Risk Factors for Long-term Disability and Work Loss*, NACHD and ACC, Wellington, 1997.

17 We also discussed one important factor that . . .: Søren Grøn et al., 'Back beliefs in patients with low back pain: a primary care cohort study', *BMC Musculoskeletal Disorders*, vol. 20, no. 1, 2019.

18 Recent research has confirmed that emotion regulation . . .: Nell Norman-Nott et al., 'Emotion regulation skills-focused interventions for chronic pain: A systematic review and meta-analysis', *European Journal of Pain*, 2024.

20 But immunologists have now realised that our . . .: Robert Dantzer, 'Neuroimmune interactions: from the brain to the immune system and vice versa', *Physiological Review*, vol. 98, no. 1, 2018, pp. 477–504.

20 Our neuroimmune system influences how we recover . . .: Micaela L. O'Reilly et al., 'Neuroimmune System as a Driving Force for Plasticity Following CNS Injury', *Frontiers in Cellular Neuroscience*, vol. 14, no. 187, 2020.

20 When we feel safe, our body optimises . . .: Stephen W. Porges, 'Polyvagal Theory: A Science of Safety', *Frontiers in Integrative Neuroscience*, vol. 16, 2022.

24 With better vagal tone comes resilience and . . .: Gabriela Guerra Leal Souza et al., 'Resilience and vagal tone predict cardiac recovery from acute social stress', *Stress*, vol. 10, no. 4, 2007, pp. 368–74.

29 Self-regulation refers to your ability to manage . . .: Roy F. Baumeister et al., *Losing control: How and why people fail at self-regulation*, Academic Press, 1994.

29 It's been found to be positively linked . . .: Surjeet Singh et al., 'Self-regulation as a correlate of psychological wellbeing', *Indian Journal of Health and Wellbeing*, vol. 9, no. 3, 2018, pp. 441–44.

30 Although self-regulation typically develops in childhood . . .: Nikki Aikens et al., 'Getting Ready for Kindergarten: Children's Progress during Head Start', *FACES*

2009 Report. Washington, DC: Office of Planning, Research and Evaluation, Administration for Children and Families, U.S. Department of Health and Human Services, 2013.

38 Constantly elevated blood pressure might also allow . . .: Bruce S. McEwen, 'Stressed or stressed out: what is the difference?', *Journal of Psychiatry and Neuroscience*, vol. 30, no. 5, 2005, pp. 315–18.

48 It also means that vital processes such . . .: Matthew J. Friedman and Bruce S. Mcewen, 'Posttraumatic Stress Disorder, Allostatic Load, and Medical Illness', Trauma and health: Physical health consequences of exposure to extreme stress, *American Psychological Association*, 2004, pp. 157–188.

38 This can amplify our sense of panic . . .: Emily R. Stern, 'Neural circuitry of interoception: new insights into anxiety and obsessive–compulsive disorders', *Current Treatment Options in Psychiatry*, vol. 1, no. 3, 2014, pp. 235–47.

39 Some studies have indicated that one of . . .: Bessel van der Kolk, *The Body Keeps the Score: Brain, Mind, and Body in the Treatment of Trauma*, Viking, New York, 2014.

39 Instead, we need to connect with our body.: Ruth A. Lanius et al., 'A review of neuroimaging studies in PTSD: heterogeneity of response to symptom provocation', *Journal of psychiatric research*, vol. 40, no. 8, 2006, pp. 709–29.

39 This sensation is very real, because when . . .: Jonathan E. Sherin et al., 'Posttraumatic stress disorder: the neurobiological impact of psychological trauma', *Dialogues in Clinical Neuroscience*, vol. 13, no. 3, 2011, pp. 263–78.

39 In one study of adults with depression . . .: Daniella J. Furman et al., 'Interoceptive awareness, positive affect, and decision making in major depressive disorder', *Journal of Affective Disorders*, vol. 151, no. 2, 2013, pp. 780–85.

40 This can be the root cause of some chronic . . .: Peter Salmon et al., 'Abuse, Dissociation, and Somatization in Irritable Bowel Syndrome: Towards an Explanatory Model', *Journal of Behavioral Medicine*, vol. 26, 2003, pp. 1–18; Robert C. Scaer, 'The neurophysiology of dissociation and chronic disease', *Applied Psychophysiology and Biofeedback*, vol. 26, no. 1, 2001, pp. 73–91; Abigail Powers et al., 'The differential effects of PTSD, MDD, and dissociation on CRP in trauma-exposed women', *Comprehensive Psychiatry*, vol. 93, 2019, 33–40; Angelo A. Alonzo, 'The experience of chronic illness and post-traumatic stress disorder: the consequences of cumulative adversity', Social Science & Medicine, vol. 50, no. 10, 2000, pp. 1475–84.

40 For example, we might not notice that . . .: Emma Goodall and Charlotte Brown, *Interoception and Regulation: Teaching Skills of Body Awareness and Supporting Connection with Others*, Jessica Kingsley Publishers, London, 2022.

48 It also means that vital processes such . . .: Meghna Ravi et al., 'The Immunology of Stress and the Impact of Inflammation on the Brain and Behavior', *BJPsych Advances*, vol. 27, no. 3, 2021, pp. 158–65; Stephen W. Porges, 'Polyvagal Theory: A Science of Safety', *Frontiers in Integrative Neuroscience*, vol. 16, 2022.

48 For example, blood pressure rises in the face . . .: Jeonogk G. Logan et al., 'Allostasis and allostatic load: expanding the discourse on stress and cardiovascular disease', *Journal of Clinical Nursing*, vol. 17, no. 7B, 2008, pp. 201–8.

50 If we spend too long in this state, we might . . .: Hanna M et al., 'Cognitive function in clinical burnout: A systematic review and meta-analysis', *Work & Stress*, vol. 36, no. 1, 2022, pp. 86–104.

55 Moving into our play state is a way . . .: Stephen W. Porges et al., *Our Polyvagal Worlds: How Safety and Trauma Change Us*, W. W. Norton & Company, 2023.

56 Sharing an intimate moment with another person . . .: ibid.

58 Fawn is a blended state that doesn't . . .: ibid.

64 This sounds like a grand promise . . .: Jenny Guidi et al., 'Allostatic load and its impact on health: a systematic review', *Psychotherapy and Psychosomatics*, vol. 90, no. 1, 2020, pp. 11–27.

64 As we've discovered this includes persistent pain . . .: Jo Nijs et al., 'The importance of stress in the paradigm shift from a tissue- and disease-based pain management approach towards multimodal lifestyle interventions for chronic pain', *Brazilian Journal of Physical Therapy*, vol. 28, no. 2, 2024; Hong-Yan Qin et al., 'Impact of psychological stress on irritable bowel syndrome', *World Journal of Gastroenterology*, vol. 20, no. 39, 2014, pp. 14126–31; Steven J. Linton, 'Does work stress predict insomnia? A prospective study', *British Journal of Health Psychology*, vol. 9, no. 2, 2010, pp. 127–36; Yun-Zi Liu et al., 'Inflammation: The Common Pathway of Stress-Related Diseases', *Frontiers in Human Neuroscience*, vol. 11, 2017.

65 Though the details behind these communication pathways . . .: Pedro Mateos-Aparicio et al., 'The Impact of Studying Brain Plasticity', *Frontiers in Cellular Neuroscience*, vol. 13, 2019.

65 Research conducted over the past two decades . . .: Babette Rothschild, *The body remembers: The psychophysiology of trauma and trauma treatment*, Norton Professional Books, New York, 2000; Linda J. Levine, 'Reconstructing memory for emotions', *Journal of Experimental Psychology: General*, vol. 126, no. 2, 1997, pp. 165–77; Pat Ogden et al., 'Sensorimotor psychotherapy: One method for processing traumatic memory', *Traumatology*, vol. 6, no. 3, 2000, pp. 149–73.

65 Though the details behind these communication pathways . . .: Pedro Mateos-Aparicio et al., 'The Impact of Studying Brain Plasticity', *Frontiers in Cellular Neuroscience*, vol. 13, 2019.

71 While we can evaluate the outer world . . .: Lisa Feldman Barrett, 'The theory of constructed emotion: an active inference account of interoception and categorization', *Social Cognitive and Affective Neuroscience*, vol. 12, no. 1, 2017, pp. 1–23.

72 In fact, 80 per cent of the . . .: Bruno Bonaz, 'The Vagus Nerve in the Neuro-Immune Axis: Implications in the Pathology of the Gastrointestinal Tract', *Frontiers in Immunology*, vol. 8, 2017.

73 If it decides we're in danger, internal alarms . . .: Stephen W. Porges, 'The polyvagal theory: New insights into adaptive reactions of the autonomic nervous system', *Cleveland Clinic Journal of Medicine*, vol. 76, no. 2, 2009.

73 Neuroception depends a lot on our past experiences . . .: Stephen W. Porges, 'Polyvagal theory: a science of safety', *Frontiers in Integrative Neuroscience*, vol. 16, 2022.

74 Adding to this cycle is the fact that we're programmed . . .: Tiffany A. Ito et al., 'Negative information weighs more heavily on the brain: the negativity bias in evaluative categorizations', *Journal of Personality and Social Psychology*, vol. 75, no. 4, 1998, pp. 887–900.

75 This can make it even harder for us to change these patterns . . .: Stephen W. Porges, 'The polyvagal theory: new insights into adaptive reactions of the autonomic nervous system', *Cleveland Clinic Journal of Medicine*, vol. 76, no. 2, 2009.

76 The interrelationship between exteroception and interoception underlies . . .: Robin Bekrater-Bodmann et al., 'Interoceptive Awareness Is Negatively Related to the Exteroceptive Manipulation of Bodily Self-Location', *Frontiers in Psychology*, vol. 11, 2020.

79 An emotion is made up of two or more bodily signals . . .: Lisa Feldman Barrett, *How Emotions Are Made: The Secret Life of the Brain*, Houghton Mifflin Harcourt, New York, 2017; Hugo D. Critchley et al., 'Interoception and emotion', *Current Opinion in Psychology*, vol. 17, 2017, pp. 7–14.

80 How we feel within ourselves based on what . . .: A. D. Craig, *How Do You Feel?: An Interoceptive Moment with Your Neurobiological Self*, Princeton University Press, New Jersey, 2015.

80 Targeting them can improve your vagal tone . . .: Thomas Pinna et al., 'A Systematic Review of Associations Between Interoception, Vagal Tone, and Emotional Regulation: Potential Applications for Mental Health, Wellbeing, Psychological Flexibility, and Chronic Conditions', *Frontiers in Psychology*, vol. 11, 2020; Archana Rajagopalan et al., 'Understanding the links between vestibular and limbic systems regulating emotions', Journal of Natural Science, Biology and Medicine, vol. 8, no. 1, 2017, pp. 11–15.

82 'An emotion is your brain's creation of what . . .': Lisa Feldman Barrett, *How Emotions Are Made: The Secret Life of the Brain*, Houghton Mifflin Harcourt, New York, 2017.

83 Within this system, electrical impulses and . . .: Leonard L. LaPointe, *Atlas of Neuroanatomy for Communication Science and Disorders*, Thieme Medical Publishers, New York, 2011.

83 There are blood vessels, of course, and . . .: Christopher S. von Bartheld, 'The Search for True Numbers of Neurons and Glial Cells in the Human Brain: A Review of 150 Years of Cell Counting', *The Journal of Comparative Neurology*, vol. 524, no. 18, 2016, pp. 3865–95.

85 Our brains didn't evolve for logical thinking . . .: Lisa Feldman Barrett, 'The theory of constructed emotion: an active inference account of interoception and categorization', *Social Cognitive and Affective Neuroscience*, vol. 12, no. 1, 2017, pp. 1–23.

85 By learning to use both of these pathways . . .: Sarah Weiss, 'On the interaction of self-regulation, interoception and pain perception', *Psychopathology*, vol. 47, no. 6, 2014, pp. 377–82.

85 It's believed that 90 per cent of brain development . . .: 'The science of early childhood development', *Bipartisan Policy Center*, 2021, bipartisanpolicy.org

85 Around age 25, the top stair forms and we reach . . .: Mariam Arain et al., 'Maturation of the adolescent brain', *Neuropsychiatric Disease and Treatment*, vol. 9, 2013, pp. 449–61.

87 Within the limbic system, the amygdala is . . .: Michael Greenwood, *Implicit vs. Explicit Memories*, 2023, www.news-medical.net

88 When we're dysregulated and experiencing strong . . .: Jaak Panksepp, *Affective Neuroscience: The Foundations of Human and Animal Emotions*, Oxford University Press, New York, 1998; Antonio R. Damasio, 'A second chance for emotion', in R.D. Lane & L. Nadel (eds), *Cognitive Neuroscience of Emotion*, Oxford University Press, New York, 2000, pp. 12–23.

88 Following trauma, specific motor areas in the survival brain . . .: Giorgio Rizzi et al., 'Excitatory rubral cells encode the acquisition of novel complex motor tasks', *Nature Communications*, vol. 10, 2019.

88 Following trauma . . . which explains why our body tightens . . .: Anna Pissota et al., 'Neurofunctional correlates of posttraumatic stress disorder: a PET symptom provocation study', *European Archives of Psychiatry and Clinical Neuroscience*, vol. 252, no. 2, 2002, pp. 68–75.

88 Also known as the cerebrum, the thinking brain . . .: Richard D. Lane et al., 'Neural substrates of conscious emotional experience: a cognitive-neuroscientific perspective', in Mario Beauregard (ed.), *Consciousness, Emotional Self-regulation and the Brain*, John Benjamins, Amsterdam, 2004, pp. 87–122; Ruth A. Lanius et al., 'A review of neuroimaging studies in PTSD: heterogeneity of response to symptom provocation', *Journal of Psychiatric Research*, vol. 40, no. 8, 2006, pp. 709–29.

90 We do this by integrating brain-down and . . .: Ann Gill Taylor et al., 'Top-Down and Bottom-Up Mechanisms in Mind-Body Medicine: Development of an Integrative Framework for Psychophysiological Research', *Explore*, vol. 6, no. 1, 2010.

90 Several studies have shown that under high levels . . .: Bessel van der Kolk, 'Posttraumatic stress disorder and the nature of trauma', *Dialogues in Clinical Neuroscience*, vol. 2, no. 1, 2000, pp. 7–22.

91 Receptors in the body also send information . . .: J. L. Taylor, 'Proprioreception', in Larry R. Squire *Encyclopedia of Neuroscience*, Academic Press, San Diego, 2009, pp. 1143–49.

92 How we perceive our body, our feelings and . . .: Nadine Gogolla, 'The insular cortex', *Current Biology*, vol. 27, no. 12, 2017.

92 By practising interoception – by using tools to . . .: A. D. (Bud) Craig, 'How do you feel — now? The anterior insula and human awareness', *Nature Reviews Neuroscience*, vol. 10, 2009, pp. 59–90.

93 In 2012, researchers released findings of a study that . . .: Martin P. Paulus et al., 'Subjecting elite athletes to inspiratory breathing load reveals behavioral and neural signatures of optimal performers in extreme environments', *PLoS One*, vol. 7, no. 1, 2012.

94 Similar observations were made during a study of elite . . .: Martin P. Paulus et al., 'Differential brain activation to angry faces by elite warfighters: neural processing evidence for enhanced threat detection', *PLoS One*, vol. 5, no. 4, 2010.

94 The authors of the study on adventure racers . . .: Martin P. Paulus et al., 'Subjecting elite athletes to inspiratory breathing load', *PLoS One*, vol. 7, no. 1, 2012.

95 As the word 'periphery' suggests, this branch of the . . .: Jill Seladi-Schulman, 'How many nerves are in the human body?', *Healthline*, 2019, www.healthline.com

103 Activating your interoceptive and peripheral nervous systems . . .: Deborah Badoud et al., 'From the body's viscera to the body's image: Is there a link between interoception and body image concerns?', *Neuroscience & Biobehavioural Reviews*, vol. 77, 2017, pp. 237–46.

105 In 1995, Dr Stephen Porges, director at the time . . .: Stephen W. Porges, 'Orienting in a defensive world: mammalian modifications of our evolutionary heritage: A polyvagal theory', *Psychophysiology*, vol. 32, no. 4, 1995, pp. 301–18.

106 This branch of the vagus nerve is myelinated.: Hisashi Hanazawa, 'Polyvagal theory and its clinical potential: an overview', *Brain and Nerve*, vol. 74, no. 8, 2022, pp. 1011–16.

109 Researchers believe that there are different groups . . .: Qiancheng Zhao et al., 'A multidimensional coding architecture of the vagal interoceptive system', *Nature*, vol. 603, no. 7903, 2022, pp. 878–84.

109 This is how the brain knows exactly who's 'calling' . . .: ibid.

110 Research has shown an association between high vagal . . .: Guy William Fincham et al., 'Effect of breathwork on stress and mental health: A meta-analysis of randomised-controlled trials', *Scientific Reports*, vol. 13, no. 1, 2023.

115 When we're in the 'too cold' dorsal vagal . . .: Gerard J. Tortora et al., *Principles of Anatomy and Physiology, 15th edition*, John Wiley & Sons, New York, 2017.

115 Without the vagal brake, the average resting . . .: Rollin McCraty et al., 'Heart Rate Variability: New Perspectives on Physiological Mechanisms, Assessment of Self-regulatory Capacity, and Health risk', *Global advances in health and medicine*, vol. 4, no. 1, 2015, pp. 46–61.

116 The re-engaging of this vagal brake is that big . . .: Stephen W. Porges, 'The vagal paradox: A polyvagal solution', *Comprehensive Psychoneuroendocrinology*, vol. 16, 2023.

120 The heart's pacemaker – the sinoatrial node . . .: Jacek Kolacz et al., 'Chronic diffuse pain and functional gastrointestinal disorders after traumatic stress: pathophysiology through a polyvagal perspective', *Frontiers in Medicine*, vol. 5, 2018.

121 Simply put, HRV is the distance between our . . .: Fred Shaffer et al., 'An overview of heart rate variability metrics and norms', *Frontiers in Public Health*, vol. 5, 2017.

121 There are wearable devices that track HRV . . .: ibid.

121 These HRV readings can provide a very . . .: Bruce S. McEwen et al., *The End of Stress as We Know It*, Joseph Henry Press, Washington, 2002; Elizabeth Stanley, *Widen the Window: Training Your Brain and Body to Thrive During Stress and Recover from Trauma*, Yellow Kite, London, 2019; Stephen W Porges, *The Polyvagal*

Theory: Neurophysiological Foundations of Emotions, Attachment, Communication, Self-regulation, W.W. Norton & Company, New York, 2011.

121 Overall, a high HRV indicates high vagal tone . . .: Thomas Pinna et al., 'A systematic review of associations between interoception, vagal tone, and emotional regulation: potential applications for mental health, wellbeing, psychological flexibility, and chronic conditions', *Frontiers in Psychology*, vol. 11, 2020; Joseph T. Marmerstein et al., 'Direct measurement of vagal tone in rats does not show correlation to HRV', *Scientific Reports*, vol. 11, no. 1, 2021.

121 Researchers consider low HRV an indication . . .: 'Heart rate variability (HRV)', *Cleveland Clinic*, 2021, my.clevelandclinic.org

122 Ideally, our heartbeat reflects the demands . . .: Rebecca Knowles et al., 'Dr. Stephen Porges' latest publication on the polyvagal theory, and what it means for the Safe and Sound Protocol (SSP)', *Unyte*, 2023, integratedlistening.com

123 Too much time in this zone can either . . .: Jacek Kolacz et al., 'Chronic diffuse pain and functional gastrointestinal disorders after traumatic stress: pathophysiology through a polyvagal perspective', *Frontiers in Medicine*, vol. 5, 2018.

125 That's because the gut, like the heart . . .: Marilia Carabotti et al., 'The gut-brain axis: interactions between enteric microbiota, central and enteric nervous systems', *Annals of Gastroenterology*, vol. 28, no. 2, 2015, pp. 203–09.

126 How much food we eat is influenced by . . .: Stephen C. Woods, 'Gastrointestinal satiety signals: I. An overview of gastrointestinal signals that influence food intake', *American Journal of Physiology. Gastrointestinal and Liver Physiology*, vol. 286, no. 1, 2004.

126 These gather information from the gut wall . . .: Melanie Maya Kaelberer et al., 'Neuropod Cells: The Emerging Biology of Gut-Brain Sensory Transduction', *Annual Review of Neuroscience*, vol. 43, 2020, pp. 337–53; Chuyue D. Yu et al., 'Vagal sensory neurons and gut-brain signalling,' *Current Opinion in Neurobiology*, vol. 62, 2020, pp. 133–140.

126 But it also helps connect the emotional and . . .: Marilia Carabotti et al., 'The gut-brain axis: interactions between enteric microbiota, central and enteric nervous systems', *Annals of Gastroenterology*, vol. 28, no. 2, 2015, pp. 203–09.

127 And when the ventral branch of the . . .: Pamela Hornby et al., 'Central control of lower esophageal sphincter relaxation', *Sensory physiology of the esophagus*, vol. 108, no. 4, 2000, pp. 90–98.

127 Promising new research shows that vagus . . .: Kun-Han Lu et al., 'Vagus nerve stimulation promotes gastric emptying by increasing pyloric opening measured with magnetic resonance imaging', *Neurogastroenterology and Motility*, vol. 30, no. 10, 2018.

127 They also produce neurotransmitters . . .: Mark Lyte, 'Microbial endocrinology in the microbiome–gut–brain axis: how bacterial production and utilization of neurochemicals influence behavior', *PLoS Pathogens*, vol. 9, no. 11, 2013.

128 These microbes are so essential to the . . .: The Nutrition Source, 'The microbiome', *Harvard T.H. Chan School of Public Health*, www.hsph.harvard.edu

128 The brain–gut–microbiota axis is . . .: Marilia Carabotti et al., 'The gut-brain axis: interactions between enteric microbiota, central and enteric nervous systems', *Annals of Gastroenterology*, vol. 28, no. 2, 2015, pp. 203–09.

128 This is why changes in this axis are often . . .: Robert P. Smith et al., 'Gut microbiome diversity is associated with sleep physiology in humans', *PLoS One*, vol. 14, no. 10, 2019.

129 This is known as gut dysbiosis . . .: Ana M. Valdes et al., 'Role of the gut microbiota in nutrition and health', *BMJ*, vol. 361, 2018.

129 As much as 70–80 per cent of our immune . . .: Selma P. Wiertsema et al., 'The interplay between the gut microbiome and the immune system in the context of infectious diseases throughout life and the role of nutrition in optimizing treatment strategies', *Nutrients*, vol. 13, no. 3, 2021.

129 The gut microbiota is essential in shaping . . .: June L. Round et al., 'The gut microbiota shapes intestinal immune responses during health and disease', *Nature Reviews. Immunology*, vol. 9, no. 5, 2009, pp. 313–23.

130 Acetylcholine slows the heart after stress . . .: Takeshi Fujii et al., 'Expression and Function of the Cholinergic System in Immune Cells', *Frontiers in Immunology*, no. 8, 2017.

131 We produce *more* ghrelin, which makes us . . .: Jean-Baptiste Bouillon-Minois et al., 'Ghrelin as a Biomarker of Stress: A Systematic Review and Meta-Analysis', *Nutrients*, vol. 13, no. 3, 2021.

134 Over time, his constipation, pain and bloating . . .: Kirsteen N. Browning et al., 'Central nervous system control of gastrointestinal motility and secretion and modulation of gastrointestinal functions', *Comprehensive Physiology*, vol. 4, no. 4, 2014, pp. 1339–68.

135 From a primal point of view, expelling . . .: Peter A. Levine, *In an Unspoken Voice: How the Body Releases Trauma and Restores Goodness*, North Atlantic, 2011.

136 Increasing vagal tone and improving his interoceptive . . .: Daniele Di Lernia et al., 'Pain in the body. Altered interoception in chronic pain conditions: A systematic review', *Neuroscience & Biobehavioral Reviews*, vol. 71, 2016, pp. 328–41; Yannick Tousignant-Laflamme et al., 'Different autonomic responses to experimental pain in IBS patients and healthy controls', *Journal of Clinical Gastroenterology*, vol. 40, no. 9, 2006, pp. 814–20.

137 The rate of anxiety is also five times higher . . .: Stephanie L. Schnorr et al., 'Integrative therapies in anxiety treatment with special emphasis on the gut microbiome', *The Yale Journal of Biology and Medicine*, vol. 89, no. 3, 2016, pp. 397–422; Arthur D. Mak et al., 'Dyspepsia is strongly associated with major depression and generalised anxiety disorder – a community study', *Alimentary Pharmacology and Therapeutics*, vol. 36, no. 8, 2012, pp.800–10; Sing Lee et al., 'Irritable bowel syndrome is strongly associated with generalized anxiety disorder: a community study', *Alimentary Pharmacology and Therapeutics*, vol. 30, no. 6, 2009, pp. 643–51.

138 Studies have indicated that engaging . . .: Simone L. Peters et al., 'Randomised clinical trial: the efficacy of gut-directed hypnotherapy is similar to that of the

low FODMAP diet for the treatment of irritable bowel syndrome', *Alimentary Pharmacology and Therapeutics*, vol. 44, no. 5, 2016, pp. 447–59.

140 Fascia extends into every structure and system . . .: Caterina Fede et al., 'Innervation of human superficial fascia', *Frontiers in Neuroanatomy*, vol. 16, 2022.

140 We have several different types of fascia . . .: 'Fascia', Physiopedia, www.physio-pedia.com

140 The deep fascia that wraps around our organs . . .: Caterina Fede et al., 'Evidence of a new hidden neural network into deep fasciae', *Scientific Reports*, vol. 11, no. 1, 2021; Robert Schleip et al., 'Interoception. A new correlate for intricate connections between fascial receptors, emotion and self recognition', *Fascia: The Tensional Network of the Human Body*, 2012, pp. 88-94.

141 Deep fascia also plays a role in proprioception . . .: Jonas Tesarz et al., 'Altered pressure pain thresholds and increased wind-up in adult patients with chronic back pain with a history of childhood maltreatment: a quantitative sensory testing study', *Pain*, vol. 157, no. 8, 2016, pp. 1799–1809.

141 This ensures our survival in the moment . . .: Paolo Tozzi, 'Does fascia hold memories?', *Journal of Bodywork and Movement Therapies*, vol. 18, no. 2, 2014, pp. 259–65.

141 Research indicates that people who have . . .: Emilio J. Puentedura, 'Combining manual therapy with pain neuroscience education in the treatment of chronic low back pain: A narrative review of the literature', *Physiotherapy theory and practice*, vol. 32, no. 5, 2016, pp. 408–14.

142 Just like we have neuroception as an . . .: A. D. (Bud) Craig, *How Do You Feel? An Interoceptive Moment with Your Neurobiological Self*, Princeton University Press, 2014.

142 And our past experience colours how we . . .: Antonio Damasioet al., 'The Nature of Feelings: Evolutionary and Neurobiological Origins.', *Nature Reviews Neuroscience*, vol. 14, no. 2, 2023, pp. 143–52.

142 Our emotions can make the pain experience . . .: Chantal Villemure et al., 'Effects of odors on pain perception: deciphering the roles of emotion and attention', *Pain*, vol. 106, no. 1–2, 2003, pp. 101–08; Katja Wiech et al., 'Neurocognitive aspects of pain perception', *Trends in Cognitive Sciences*, vol. 12, no. 8, 2008, pp. 306–313.

144 When we work with our fascia, we . . .: Robert Schleip, 'Fascial plasticity – a new neurobiological explanation: Part 1', *Journal of Bodywork and Movement Therapies*, vol. 7, no. 1, 2003, pp. 11–19.

145 Phantom limb pain, which is when we . . .: R. Melzack, 'Phantom limbs and the concept of a neuromatrix', *Trends in Neurosciences*, vol. 13, no. 3, 1990, p. 88–92; Amreet Kaur et al., 'Phantom limb pain: A literature review', *Chinese Journal of Traumatology*, vol. 21, no. 6, 2018, pp. 336–68.

146 The pain not only feels real, but . . .: R. Melzack et al., 'Phantom limbs in people with congenital limb deficiency or amputation in early childhood', *Brain: Journal of Neurology*, vol. 120, no. 9, 1997, pp. 1603–20.

148 Sensations, whether they are overwhelming bodily signals . . .: John A. Sturgeon et al., 'Social pain and physical pain: shared paths to resilience', *Pain Management*, vol. 6, no. 1, 2016, pp. 63–74.

147 The pain from that one finger might . . .: Lorimer Moseley et al., 'Targeting cortical representations in the treatment of chronic pain: a review', *Neurorehabilitation and Neural Repair*, vol. 26, no. 6, 2012, pp. 646–52.

151 Neuroplasticity is the incredible ability of neural . . .: Moheb Costandi, *Neuroplasticity*, The MIT Press, 2016.

158 These three areas of the body communicate . . .: Stephen W. Porges, 'Polyvagal Theory: A Science of Safety', *Frontiers in Integrative Neuroscience*, vol. 16, 2022.

158 When we're around someone who is experiencing . . .: Daniel J. Siegel, *Mindsight: Change Your Brain And Your Life*, Scribe Publications, 2012; Stephen W. Porges, 'Social Engagement and Attachment: A Phylogenetic Perspective', *Annuals of the New York Academy of Sciences*, vol. 1008, 2003, pp. 31–47.

159 This allows us to flee danger, find . . .: ibid.

160 Feeling lonely or isolated can cause distress . . .: J. T. Cacioppo et al., 'Lonely traits and concomitant physiological processes: the MacArthur social neuroscience studies', *International Journal of Psychophysiology*, vol. 32, no. 2–3, 2000, pp. 143–154; Michaela Reimers et al., 'Rehabilitation of research chimpanzees: stress and coping after long-term isolation', *Hormones and Behavior*, vol. 51, no. 3, 2007, pp. 428–35.

160 If left unchecked, these can lead to . . .: LaBarron K. Hill et al., 'The Autonomic Nervous System and Hypertension: Ethnic Differences and Psychosocial Factors', *Current cardiology reports*, vol. 21, no. 3, 2019; R. D. Brook et al., 'Autonomic imbalance, hypertension, and cardiovascular risk', *American Journal of Hypertension*, vol. 13, no. 6, 2000.

160 In fact, feeling that you belong and having . . .: Yang Claire Yang et al., 'Social relationships and physiological determinants of longevity across the human life span', *Proceedings of the National Academy of Sciences of the United States of America*, vol. 113, no. 3, 2016, pp. 578–83.

160 Research shows that supportive social . . .: V. R. Venna et al. 'Social interaction plays a critical role in neurogenesis and recovery after stroke', *Translational Psychiatry*, vol. 4, no. 1, 2014.

160 Strengthening your own relational web and . . .: Ruth Feldman, 'Social behavior as a transdiagnostic marker of resilience', *Annual Review of Clinical Psychology*, vol. 17, 2021, pp. 153–80.

161 When we use the safety signals others . . .: Marc H. Bornstein et al., 'Coregulation: a multilevel approach via biology and behavior', *Children*, vol. 10, no. 8, 2023.

161 The relationships we have with the people . . .: L. Alan Sroufe, Early relationships and the development of children, *Infant Mental Health Journal*, vol. 21, pp. 67–74, 2000.

161 This goes both ways, too: the child's distress . . .: Richard Chambers et al., 'Mindful emotion regulation: an integrative review', *Clinical Psychology Review*, vol. 29, no. 6, 2009, pp. 560–72.

161 This process, while it may seem instinctual . . .: Allan Schore, *Affect Regulation and the Origin of the Self: The Neurobiology of Emotional Development*, Lawrence Erlbaum Associates, New Jersey, 1994.

161 In the same way a house's plumbing and . . .: ibid.

163 Empirical research has shown how leaders and . . .: Janne Skakon et al., 'Are leaders' well-being, behaviours and style associated with the affective well-being of their employees? A systematic review of three decades of research', *Work & Stress*, vol. 24, no. 2, 2010, pp. 107–39.

163 We know that if we lack a connection . . .: Emma Goodall and Charlotte Brown, 2022, op. cit.

176 Remember, 80 per cent of the messages whizzing . . .: Sara L. Prescott et al., 'Internal senses of the vagus nerve', *Neuron*, vol. 110, no. 4, 2022, pp. 579–99.

177 When we introduce a new experience . . .: Alessandro Sale et al., 'Environment and brain plasticity: towards an endogenous pharmacotherapy', *Physiological Reviews*, vol. 94, no. 1, 2014, pp. 189–234.

177 If you've heard of placebo effect . . .: David Spiegel et al., 'What is the placebo worth?', *BMJ*, vol. 336, no. 7651, 2008, pp. 967–68.

178 These drivers hadn't been born with enlarged . . .: Eleanor A. Maguire et al., 'Navigation-related structural change in the hippocampi of taxi drivers', *Proceedings of the National Academy of Sciences*, vol. 97, no. 8, 2000.

178 The term 'bioplasticity' was coined by physiotherapist . . .: Mick Thacker et al., 'First-person neuroscience and the understanding of pain', *The Medical Journal of Australia*, vol. 196, no. 6, 2012, pp. 410–11.

179 Children's earliest years are considered the 'golden years' . . .: Catherine Morgan, 'Harnessing neuroplasticity to improve motor performance in infants with cerebral palsy: a study protocol for the GAME randomised controlled trial', *BMJ Open*, vol. 13, no. 3, 2023.

186 The science suggests that too much . . .: Wolf Mehling, 'Differentiating attention styles and regulatory aspects of self-reported interoceptive sensibility', *Philosophical transactions of the Royal Society of London. Series B, Biological sciences*, vol. 371, no. 1708, 2016.

195 It bears repeating that one of the . . .: ibid.

213 If, for example, you're stuck in a dorsal . . .: Paul A. Frewen et al., 'Toward a psychobiology of posttraumatic self-dysregulation: reexperiencing, hyperarousal, dissociation, and emotional numbing', *Annals of the New York Academy of Sciences*, vol. 1071, 2006, pp. 110–24; James W. Hopper et al., 'Neural correlates of reexperiencing, avoidance, and dissociation in PTSD: symptom dimensions and emotion dysregulation in responses to script-driven trauma imagery', *Journal of Traumatic Stress*, vol. 20, no. 5, 2007, pp. 713–25; Ruth A. Lanius et al., 'Functional connectivity of dissociative responses in posttraumatic stress disorder: a functional magnetic resonance imaging investigation', *Biological Psychiatry*, vol. 57, no. 8, 2005, pp. 873–84; Erika J. Wolf et al., 'The dissociative subtype of PTSD: a replication and extension', *Depression and anxiety*, vol. 29,

no. 8, 2012, pp. 679–88; Ulrich F. Lanius et al. (eds), *Neurobiology and Treatment of Traumatic Dissociation: Towards an Embodied Self*, Springer Publishing, New York, 2014.

218 Slow breathing, for example, results . . .: Pierre Philippot et al., 'Respiratory feedback in the generation of emotion', *Cognition and Emotion*, vol. 16, no. 5, 2002, pp. 605–27.

218 Research indicates that practising daily . . .: V. C. Goessl et al., 'The effect of heart rate variability biofeedback training on stress and anxiety: a meta-analysis', *Psychological Medicine*, vol. 47, no. 15, 2017, pp. 2578–86; Paul Lehrer et al., 'Heart rate variability biofeedback improves emotional and physical health and performance: a systematic review and meta analysis', *Applied Psychophysiology and Biofeedback*, vol. 45, 2020, pp. 109–29; Silvia F. M. Pizzoli et al., 'A meta-analysis on heart rate variability biofeedback and depressive symptoms', *Scientific Reports*, vol. 11, no. 1, 2021.

223 If an antelope that outruns a lion . . .: Richard Chambers et al., 'Mindful emotion regulation: an integrative review', *Clinical Psychology Review*, vol. 29, no. 6, 2009, pp. 560–72.

227 People with high emotional granularity . . .: Lisa Feldman Barrett et al., 'Knowing what you're feeling and knowing what to do about it: mapping the relation between emotion differentiation and emotion regulation', *Cognition and Emotion*, vol. 15, no. 6, 2001, pp. 713–24; Elise K. Kalokerinos et al., 'Differentiate to regulate: low negative emotion differentiation is associated with ineffective use but not selection of emotion-regulation strategies', *Psychological Science*, vol. 30, no. 6, 2019, pp. 863–79.

230 Since even complex emotions begin as sensations . . .: Peter Payne et al., 'Somatic experiencing: using interoception and proprioception as core elements of trauma therapy', *Frontiers in Psychology*, vol. 6, 2015; Bessel A can der Kolk, 'Clinical implications of neuroscience research in PTSD', *Annuals of the New York Academy of Sciences*, vol. 1071, 2006, pp. 277–93; Stephen W. Porges, 'The polyvagal theory: New insights into adaptive reactions of the autonomic nervous system', *Cleveland Clinic Journal of Medicine*, vol. 76, no. 2, 2009.

236 Light touch has been shown to activate . . .: Laura Crucianelli et al., 'Interoception as independent cardiac, thermosensory, nociceptive, and affective touch perceptual submodalities', *Biological Psychology*, vol. 172, 2022.

239 If movement is challenging for you because . . .: J Schwoebel et al., 'Pain and the body schema: effects of pain severity on mental representations of movement', *Neurology*, vol. 59, no. 5, 2002.

239 Sound therapy has been shown to . . .: Nadia Rajabalee et al., 'Neuromodulation Using Computer-Altered Music to Treat a Ten-Year-Old Child Unresponsive to Standard Interventions for Functional Neurological Disorder', *Harvard Review of Psychiatry*, vol. 30, no. 5, 2022.

239 In one study, it was associated with . . .: Lucy Warhurst et al., 'Listen to your heart: a preliminary investigation of the impact of sound therapy on heart rate variability',

poster presented at the 22nd Australasian Psychophysiology Conference, *University of New South Wales*, Sydney, 2012.

244 Stretching of baroreceptors as a result of . . .: Otto Appenzeller et. al., 'Chapter 5 – Pain perception and the autonomic nervous system', *Introduction to Clinical Aspects of the Autonomic Nervous System (Sixth Edition)*, Academic Press, 2022, Pages 109–135.

245 Recent research has also shown how it . . .: Hsin-Yung Chen et al., 'Physiological Effects of Deep Touch Pressure on Anxiety Alleviation: The Weighted Blanket Approach', *Journal of Medical and Biological Engineering*, vol. 33, no. 5, 2013, pp. 463–70.

264 As we saw in Chapter 8, research tells us . . .: Alison Pearce Stevens, 'Music has the power to move us physically and emotionally. Here's why', 1 February 2024, www.snexplores.org

259 This tool recruits your complex and potentially . . .: Matthew K. Bagg et al., 'Effect of Graded Sensorimotor Retraining on Pain Intensity in Patients With Chronic Low Back Pain: A Randomized Clinical Trial', *JAMA*, vol. 328, no. 5, 2022, pp. 430–39.

259 If you have the tolerance, you can . . .: Hsin-Yung Chen et al., 2013, op. cit.

260 This is a wonderful way to 'train' . . .: Bruno Bonaz et al., 'Diseases, Disorders, and Comorbidities of Interoception', *Trends in Neurosciences*, vol. 44, no. 1, 2021, pp. 39–51.

266 Research tells us that anxiety and depression . . .: 'What is anxiety?', *Psychology Today*, www.psychologytoday.com; 'What is depression?', *Psychology Today*, www.psychologytoday.com

293 As babies, the way we are born . . .: Marta Reyman et al., 'Impact of delivery mode-associated gut microbiota dynamics on health in the first year of life', *Nature Communications*, vol. 10, 2019; Maria Dominguez-Bello et al., 'Delivery mode shapes the acquisition and structure of the initial microbiota across multiple body habitats in newborns', *Proceedings of the National Academy of Sciences of the United State of America*, vol. 107, 2010; Albert M. Levin et al., 'Joint effects of pregnancy, sociocultural, and environmental factors on early life gut microbiome structure and diversity', *Scientific Reports*, vol. 6, 2016; Martin F. Laursen et al., 'First foods and gut microbes', *Frontiers in Microbiology*, vol. 8, 2017.

293 The environment we live in, the people . . .: Meghan B. Azad et al., 'Infant gut microbiota and the hygiene hypothesis of allergic disease: impact of household pets and siblings on microbiota composition and diversity', *Allergy, asthma, and clinical immunology: official journal of the Canadian Society of Allergy and Clinical Immunology*, vol. 9, no. 1, 2013.

293 It can also change drastically depending . . .: Megan Cully, 'Antibiotics alter the gut microbiome and host health', *Nature Portfolio*, 2019, www.nature.com

295 These ingredients can be considered . . .: Mohammed Abu Tayab et al., 'Targeting neuroinflammation by polyphenols: A promising therapeutic approach against inflammation-associated depression', *Biomedicine & Pharmacotherapy*, vol. 147, 2022.

295 While there's no blueprint for the perfect . . .: Ana M. Valdes et al., 'Role of the gut microbiota in nutrition and health', *BMJ*, vol. 361, 2018.

295 Given the relationship between the gut . . .: ibid.

296 Processed foods increase inflammation . . .: Chieh-Hsin Lee et al., 'The role of inflammation in depression and fatigue', *Frontiers in Immunology*, vol. 10, 2019.

296 In the landmark SMILEs trial, researchers . . .: Felice N. Jacka et al., 'A randomised controlled trial of dietary improvement for adults with major depression (the 'SMILES' trial)', *BMC Medicine*, vol. 15, no. 1, 2017.

296 This finding has been replicated in . . .: 'The SMILEs Trial', *Food and Mood*, foodandmoodcentre.com.au

296 Numerous studies have associated taking . . .: Rebecca Frances Slykerman et al., 'Effect of Lactobacillus rhamnosus HN001 in pregnancy on postpartum symptoms of depression and anxiety: a randomised double-blind placebo-controlled trial', *EBioMedicine*, vol. 24, 2017, pp. 159–65.

296–97 Numerous studies . . . to alleviating anxiety symptoms in chronic . . .: A. Venket Rao et al., 'A randomized, double-blind, placebo-controlled pilot study of a probiotic in emotional symptoms of chronic fatigue syndrome', *Gut Pathogens*, vol. 1, no. 1, 2009.

296–97 Numerous studies . . . and improving cortisol regulation, immune . . .: Asma Kazemi et al., 'Effect of prebiotic and probiotic supplementation on circulating pro-inflammatory cytokines and urinary cortisol levels in patients with major depressive disorder: a double-blind, placebo-controlled randomized clinical trial', *Journal of Functional Foods*, vol. 52, 2019, pp. 596–602; Colin Hill et al., 'Expert consensus document. The International Scientific Association for Probiotics and Prebiotics consensus statement on the scope and appropriate use of the term probiotic', *Nature reviews. Gastroenterology & hepatology*, vol. 11, 2014, pp. 506–14.

298 This enhances immunity, helps the body . . .: M. B. Geuking et al., 'The interplay between the gut microbiota and the immune system', *Gut Microbes*, vol. 5, no.3, 2014, pp. 411–418.

299 When it comes to treating depression . . .: Ben Singh et al., 'Effectiveness of physical activity interventions for improving depression, anxiety and distress: an overview of systematic reviews', *British Journal of Sports Medicine*, vol. 57, no. 18, 2023, pp. 1203–09.

299 That's not to say that counselling and . . .: 'Exercise more effective than medicines to manage mental health', *University of South Australia*, 2023, www.unisa.edu.au

299 [bullet list]: . . . improves the normal functioning of the immune system: Richard J. Simpson et al., 'Chapter Fifteen – Exercise and the regulation of immune functions', *Progress in Molecular Biology and Translational Science*, vol. 135, 2015, pp. 355–80.

299 [bullet list]: . . . has a positive influence on the endocrine system . . .: Derek Ball, 'Metabolic and endocrine response to exercise: sympathoadrenal integration with skeletal muscle', *Journal of Endocrinology*, vol. 224, no. 2, 2015.

299 [bullet list]: . . . helps control blood sugar levels, metabolism . . .: Matthieu Clauss et al., 'Interplay between exercise and gut microbiome in the context of human health and performance', *Frontiers in Nutrition*, vol. 8, 2021.

299 [bullet list]: . . . enhances cardiac function by increasing heart rate . . .: R. Hambrecht et al., 'Regular Physical Activity Improves Endothelial Function in Patients with Coronary Artery Disease by Increasing Phosphorylation of Endothelial Nitric Oxide Synthase', *Circulation*, vol. 107, no. 25, 2003.

300 [bullet list]: . . . reduces adrenaline levels at rest . . .: 'Exercise Endocrine System Interaction', *Physiopedia*, 27 Aug 2022, www.physio-pedia.com

300 [bullet list]: . . . increases serotonin levels, which can positively . . .: ibid.

300 [bullet list]: . . . memory: 'Memory', *Physiopedia*, www.physio-pedia.com

300 [bullet list]: . . . and sleep: 'Sleep: theory, function and physiology', *Physiopedia*, www.physio-pedia.com

300 [bullet list]: positively influences gut microbiota: Matthieu Clauss et al., 'Interplay Between Exercise and Gut Microbiome in the Context of Human Health and Performance', *Frontiers in Nutrition*, vol. 8, 2021.

301 Often, friends and family tell us to . . .: Nicole Emma Andrews et al., '"It's very hard to change yourself": an exploration of overactivity in people with chronic pain using interpretative phenomenological analysis', *Pain*, vol. 156, no. 7, 2015, pp. 1215–31; Nicole E. Andrews et al., 'Activity pacing, avoidance, endurance, and associations with patient functioning in chronic pain: a systematic review and meta-analysis', *Archives of Physical Medicine and Rehabilitation*, vol. 93, no. 11, 2012, pp. 2109–21.

301 Pushing harder often leads to pain flares . . .: Nicole Emma Andrews et al., '"It's very hard to change yourself": an exploration of overactivity in people with chronic pain using interpretative phenomenological analysis', *Pain*, vol. 156, no. 7, 2015, pp. 1215–31.

301 Pushing harder . . . and avoiding activity completely . . .: Nicole E. Andrews et al., 'Activity pacing, avoidance, endurance, and associations with patient functioning in chronic pain: a systematic review and meta-analysis', *Archives of Physical Medicine and Rehabilitation*, vol. 93, no. 11, 2012, pp. 2109–21.

302 If a condition such as fibromyalgia, persistent pain . . .: Rena Gatzounis et al., 'Operant learning theory in pain and chronic pain rehabilitation', *Current Pain and Headache Reports*, vol. 16, no. 2, 2012, pp. 117–26; Mélanie Racine et al., 'Operant Learning Versus Energy Conservation Activity Pacing Treatments in a Sample of Patients with Fibromyalgia Syndrome: A Pilot Randomized Controlled Trial', *The Journal of Pain*, vol. 20, no. 4, 2019.

302 Pacing is important in pain management . . .: Nicole E. Andrews et al., 'Activity pacing, avoidance, endurance, and associations with patient functioning in chronic pain: a systematic review and meta-analysis', *Archives of Physical Medicine and Rehabilitation*, vol. 93, no. 11, 2012, pp. 2109–21; Warren R. Nielson et al., 'A content analysis of activity pacing in chronic pain: what are we measuring and why?', *The Clinical Journal of Pain*, vol. 30, no. 7, 2014, pp. 639–45.

305 From a co-regulation perspective, time spent with . . .: 'Having a dog can help your heart — literally', Harvard Health Publishing, Harvard Medical School, 1 September 2015, www.health.harvard.edu

305 Dogs in particular have been linked . . .: Digestive Disease Week, 'Living with dogs (but not cats) as a toddler might protect against Crohn's disease', *ScienceDaily*, 2022, www.sciencedaily.com

305 [bullet list]: Co-regulation: Interacting with a therapy . . .: Emily L. R. Thelwell, 'Paws for thought: a controlled study investigating the benefits of interacting with a house-trained dog on university students mood and anxiety', *Animals*, vol. 9, no. 10, 2019.

305 [bullet list]: Animal-intervention programs in hospitals . . .: Fabrizio Bert et al., 'Animal assisted intervention: a systematic review of benefits and risks', European Journal of Integrative Medicine, vol. 8, no. 5, 2016, pp. 695–706.

306 [bullet list]: interoceptive accuracy: movement . . .: Amie Wallman-Jones et al., 'How physical activity can help you listen to your body', *Frontiers for Young Minds*, 2022, kids.frontiersin.org

306 [bullet list]: exteroception: targeting our tactile . . .: Debbie J. Silkwood-Sherer et al., 'Hippotherapy – an intervention to habilitate balance deficits in children with movement disorders: a clinical trial', *Physical Therapy*, vol. 92, no. 5, 2012, pp. 707–17; Danielle Champagne et al., 'Improving gross motor function and postural control with hippotherapy in children with Down syndrome: case reports', *Physiotherapy Theory and Practice*, vol. 26, no. 8, 2010, pp. 564–71; Dorothée Debuse et al., 'An exploration of German and British physiotherapists' views on the effects of hippotherapy and their measurement', *Physiotherapy Theory and Practice*, vol. 21, no. 4, 2005, pp. 219–42.

307 It impacts the ventral vagal state which . . .: Stephen M. James et al., 'Shift work: disrupted circadian rhythms and sleep – implications for health and well-being', *Current Sleep Medicine Reports*, vol. 3, 2017, pp. 104–12; Daniela Grimaldi et al., 'Adverse impact of sleep restriction and circadian misalignment on autonomic function in healthy young adults', *Hypertension*, vol. 68, no. 1, 2016, pp. 243–50.

Notes